ALLERGY-PROOF
YOUR LIFE

ALLERGY-PROOF YOUR LIFE

NATURAL REMEDIES FOR
ALLERGIES THAT WORK!

MICHELLE SCHOFFRO COOK,
PhD, DNM, ROHP

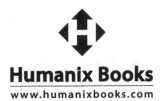

Humanix Books
www.humanixbooks.com

Humanix Books

Allergy-Proof Your Life
Copyright © 2017 by Humanix Books

Humanix Books, P.O. Box 20989, West Palm Beach, FL 33416, USA
www.humanixbooks.com | info@humanixbooks.com

Library of Congress Cataloging-in-Publication Data

Names: Cook, Michelle Schoffro, author.
Title: Allergy-proof your life : natural remedies for allergies that work! / Michelle
    Schoffro Cook, PhD, DNM, ROHP.
Other titles: Allergy proof your life
Description: Palm Beach, FL : Humanix Books, [2017] | Includes index. |
    Description based on print version record and CIP data provided by pub-
    lisher; resource not viewed.
Identifiers: LCCN 2016038180 (print) | LCCN 2016035426 (ebook) | ISBN
    9781630060756 (e-book) | ISBN 9781630060749 (hardback) | ISBN
    978163006-0756 (Ebook)
Subjects: LCSH: Allergy—Prevention. | BISAC: HEALTH & FITNESS /
    Allergies.
Classification: LCC RC584 (print) | LCC RC584 .C64 2017 (ebook) | DDC
    616.97—dc23
LC record available at https://lccn.loc.gov/2016038180

Interior Design: Scribe Inc.

Humanix Books is a division of Humanix Publishing, LLC. Its trademark, con-
sisting of the word "Humanix," is registered in the Patent and Trademark Office
and in other countries.

Disclaimer: The information presented in this book is meant to be used for general
resource purposes only; it is not intended as specific medical advice for any individual and should not substitute medical advice from a healthcare professional.
If you have (or think you may have) a medical problem, speak to your doctor or
healthcare practitioner immediately about your risk and possible treatments. Do
not engage in any therapy or treatment without consulting a medical professional.

ISBN: 978-1-63006-074-9 (Hardcover)
ISBN: 978-1-63006-075-6 (E-book)

Printed in the United States of America
10 9 8 7 6 5 4 3 2 1

Dedication

I dedicate this book to the love of my life, Curtis. You always were and always will be my one and only love.

And to my wonderful parents, Michael and Deborah Schoffro, thank for your constant belief in me as well as your love and encouragement to fulfill my dream of helping people through my writing.

Acknowledgments

TO THE MANY WONDERFUL people who helped make this book happen, including:

Curtis Cook, the love of my life, my husband, and my soulmate. I am eternally grateful for your love and am so thrilled to spend my life with you. Thank you for your constant care, love, friendship, and support. There is no better man than you.

Claire Gerus, thank you. You are a visionary agent and a great friend. I appreciate your ongoing efforts to secure my books and your many insights throughout my career.

Mary Glenn and Debra Englander, thanks for your support of my work and vision for this book. I appreciate it.

Michael and Deborah Schoffro, thank you, Mom and Dad. You have always been wonderful parents and so supportive of my writing. Thank you for your encouragement and love.

To the team at Humanix, thanks for your many efforts to bring this book to those people suffering from allergies, asthma, sinusitis, and rhinitis.

Josephine Mariea, you're a rare editor who can balance editing with maintaining the author's voice. Thank you for walking that fine line and being a real pleasure to work with.

Contents

INTRODUCTION

What Your Doctor Isn't Telling You *Is* Hurting You!

BEFORE YOU HEAD TO your doctor for painful allergy shots or pop your next antihistamine pill, I want to share some exciting news with you: *you don't have to simply suffer from allergies or mask allergy symptoms with invasive shots and harsh drugs.* More and more research shows that you can significantly reduce your allergies, not just the uncomfortable symptoms of allergies, through specific foods, nutrients, herbs, therapies, and other natural approaches.

That's great news for anyone who has been suffering from the many uncomfortable and sometimes disabling symptoms of allergies. Let's face it: if you love the outdoors, pollen, mold, and other allergies can make your life downright miserable. And then there are the indoor allergen-causing substances like dust, dust mites, animal dander, and more. I'm going to share some of the most exciting research along with my antiallergy diet and lifestyle approach that will help get your health back, enabling you to enjoy the hobbies or work you enjoy and boosting your overall quality of life.

According to the Centers for Disease Control and Prevention (CDC), an estimated 19.1 million adults in the United States were diagnosed with hay fever just in the last year.[1] An additional 6.1 million children experienced hay fever symptoms in the last year alone. On top of that, 7.4 million children had respiratory allergies and still another 8.5 million kids had skin allergies in the last year alone.[2] That's a lot of sneezing, congestion, itching and hives, and trouble breathing.

Although drugs may temporarily relieve some of the aggravating symptoms, the flip side is potentially serious: the list of side effects can be worse than the condition itself. Most people don't realize there are many natural options to alleviating allergies, including ones that are far superior to the drug options. Many doctors could recommend natural options, but few even know which ones to prescribe. Sadly, most medical doctors still don't receive any training in the use of food as medicine, herbal medicine, or nutrient supplementation. And as drug companies continue to market drugs as the exclusive options for people suffering from allergies, physicians continue to prescribe them in droves.

Before we discuss the options available to you, let's first consider: What exactly are *allergies*? According to the *Oxford Dictionary*, allergies are "a damaging immune response by the body to a substance, especially pollen, fur, a particular food, or dust, to which it has become hypersensitive."[3] But what causes the immune response to go haywire? Even as scientists continue to search for causal factors, there are numerous reasons that have been found, including a leaky gut, nutritional deficiencies, low-grade inflammation in the gut or throughout the body, and excessive sugar and dairy consumption, to name a few.

Our Standard American Diet (SAD) seems to contribute to the prevalence of allergies; switching to a low-allergen, mucusless, and clean diet seems to dramatically transform allergies in many people. I've witnessed this result personally with countless patients, some of whose stories I will share in this book.

Nutrient deficiencies also seem to contribute to weakened systems in the body and to allergy symptoms, and they may actually be a major factor in whether allergies occur at all.

Poor gut health—including microbial imbalances, insufficient allergy-reducing probiotics, inflammation, and a leaky gut—also seems to play a significant role in allergies.

Excessive stress, insufficient activity, and energy blockages throughout the body can also contribute to weakness and susceptibility to allergies in many people.

But it is insufficient to simply know the factors that play a role in causing allergies; you also need to know how to address them. A diagnosis by your doctor and a prescription for pharmaceutical drugs or allergy shots is also insufficient, as none of these options tell you why you're suffering from allergies in the first place. You need to get to the bottom of your allergies so you can correct the imbalances involved with causing them and, ultimately, reverse them in part or altogether.

Allergy-Proof Your Life: Natural Remedies for Allergies That Work! offers you an opportunity to discover your body's potential underlying weaknesses—such as nutritional deficiencies, bodily imbalances, and lifestyle choices—so you can get to the bottom of what's causing the allergies in your body—and get rid of them! Addressing the root causes of allergies is much more effective than taking a drug-based Band-Aid approach that merely lessens symptoms and worsens health in the long term.

When it comes to allergies, what your doctor doesn't know *is* hurting you. *Allergy-Proof Your Life* works by resetting your natural body chemistry and addressing the underlying causal factors for allergies instead of the medical approach to reducing symptoms at a high cost to the body. As you will soon discover, cutting-edge research shows that low-grade inflammation, nutritional deficiencies, a leaky or inflamed gut, and an inflammatory diet puts you at risk of experiencing allergies or aggravating existing allergies.

In *Allergy-Proof Your Life*, I will reveal how you can eat to beat inflammation, identify foods that contribute to environmental and seasonal allergies and foods that heal them, reverse nutritional deficiencies, and heal the gut imbalances that are frequently at the root of allergies. Sadly, that's probably not something your doctor has ever told you.

You'll find dozens of cutting-edge, scientifically proven natural therapies and remedies for allergies that have never before been compiled into a single book and many of which are virtually unknown—the product of my twenty-five years of research and experience in the natural health field. I am a registered nutritionist, board-certified doctor of natural medicine, certified herbalist, doctor of acupuncture, and the author of nineteen other natural health books. I spend almost every day researching the best proven natural medicines to help people overcome illnesses they may believe are incurable. My quest to offer the best healing advice for the treatment of allergies and other health problems has led me to research new and advanced natural treatments, including potent phytonutrients—plant nutrients—that combat symptoms, enzyme therapy to address inflammation and allergy symptoms, and orthomolecular therapy that addresses the causal factors of the condition. My clients and readers alike regularly share their successes in transforming their health and improving their quality of life.

I compiled this information into one book in my quest to empower you to take charge of your life and to put health and healing information into a practical, do-it-yourself format that is easy to follow and use. It is my hope that you will experience a health transformation.

In chapter 1, you'll learn more about the medical view of allergies as compared to a holistic one and explore some of the dangers of common allergy medications. Chapter 1 also examines the most common medications for allergies, including antihistamines, decongestants, and corticosteroids, along with the serious side effects of each. It explains why these drugs are high risk and low reward. I explore the limitations of taking a drug-based approach to allergies and why this approach won't work in the long run. I introduce the value of a holistic approach to allergies and its benefits. In chapter 2, you'll discover the most common foods that cause or worsen allergies and aggravate sinus, skin, respiratory, or other symptoms as well foods that contain natural antihistamine compounds that you can add to your diet to help boost your body's innate healing capacity. You'll also learn about the sugar and dairy connection to allergies along with the best carbs to eat. You'll discover the best antiallergy foods that can help you on your path to health. You'll explore my antiallergy diet that I developed over more than two decades and working with thousands of clients. In chapter 3, you'll uncover a little-known nutritional cause of allergies and how correcting the gut's link to allergy symptoms not only can have a huge impact on symptoms but may also even halt the condition in its tracks. It explains how correcting bacterial imbalances and a leaky gut can stop allergies in their tracks. This chapter tells you how to benefit from the exciting but little-known research. In chapter 4, you'll discover the enzymes that literally dissolve mucus and quell inflammation. Exciting research shows that systemic enzyme therapy is the natural medicine of the future when it comes to many conditions, including allergies. This chapter will detail the most exciting research, explain what it means for you, and guide you to incorporate this newfound enzyme therapy knowledge with great healing results. In chapter 5, you'll learn about natural medicines that work to reverse allergies and their many symptoms—from specific nutrients like quercetin and herbs like perilla or butterbur, among others. You'll learn about the best nutrients, what works, what works but only in specific instances, what doesn't work, and how to benefit from some of the popular natural remedies that have been found to be effective against allergies as well as many other botanical and nutritional remedies. I guide you on selecting the best remedies for you and instructs you on the dose to take and the way to take them for the best results. In chapter 6, you'll discover the many great acupressure points that have been proven effective for alleviating the symptoms of allergies. Regardless of whether you're suffering from congestion, sneezing, sinus swelling, or other allergic symptoms, you'll learn how to use the healing power in your fingertips to stop suffering! If you think aromatherapy is just about baths and spa treatments, you'll be pleasantly surprised to learn in chapter 7 that a form of medical aromatherapy, which goes well beyond the bath and beauty industry's interpretation of this science, is showing huge promise against allergy symptoms. Medical aromatherapy— a scientific approach to aromatherapy that uses the potent natural chemical constituents found in key essential oils—has been proven to have potent antihistamine effects, encourage drainage of the sinuses, boost energy, and more. You'll discover the best essential oils for allergies and learn how to use them for maximum relief. In chapter 8, you'll learn about other therapies and natural approaches to allergies that will improve your quality of life. You'll also learn how exposure to certain household and body care products may unwittingly be aggravating your allergies, worsening your breathing, or contributing to your other symptoms. And finally, in chapter 9, you'll enjoy delicious and nutritious healing recipes that can help you integrate allergy-soothing foods into your day-to-day life. From juices and teas to main dishes and even desserts, eating for healing never tasted so good. It includes recipes like Antihistamine Juice, GI Soothing Tea, Roasted Vegetable and Rosemary Soup, Mixed Berry

Pie, and Almond-Oat Thumbprint Cookies. You'll also discover recipes for making your own All-Natural All-Purpose Cleaner, Natural Glass Cleaner, Natural Laundry Soap, and other household cleaning products to avoid chemical ones that are probably aggravating your allergies.

Allergy-Proof Your Life offers you a wide variety of both cutting-edge and tried-and-true natural therapies without the harmful side effects of common antihistamine, decongestant, and corticosteroid drugs. It offers you all the tools you'll need to enjoy allergy-free living and an improved quality of life.

1

A Medical and Holistic View of Allergies

IF YOU SUFFER FROM the wide array of seasonal allergy symptoms such as fatigue; sinus congestion; itchy eyes, nose, or throat; or watery eyes, don't let a high pollen count, mold-laden leaf debris, or another allergen get you down. There are many all-natural solutions that have helped others improve and even eliminate their allergy symptoms altogether.

No one knows exactly why an everyday substance is harmless to one person and why another person's immune system wages war on the substance when he or she comes in contact with it, but there are many natural approaches that work wonders at restoring a balanced immune response. Whether tree pollens, animal dander, dust mites, or other environmental allergens, once they are inhaled or ingested, the body signals the immune system to destroy the offenders. In doing so, your cells release histamine and other chemicals, causing the classic itchy eyes, scratchy throat, runny nose, sinus congestion, or headache, among other symptoms.

Although the medical approach is to take antihistamines, most have side effects like drowsiness or can aggravate heart arrhythmias, not to mention that they are only treating the symptoms, not getting to the cause of the allergies. Let's explore some of the main medical approaches to treating allergies, along with the side effects they cause.

WHAT EXACTLY ARE ALLERGIES?

Spring allergies affect an estimated 25 million Americans.[1] Caused by an immune system overreaction to airborne pollens or other substances, spring allergies are commonly called seasonal allergies, hay fever, or allergic rhinitis.

Your immune system is your body's defense against foreign invaders; it works hard to protect you against bacteria, fungi, yeasts, viruses, toxins, and other substances that may compromise your health. We simply could not live without a strong immune system, but sometimes this impressive internal system can go a bit haywire, reacting to common, everyday substances.

Allergies are caused by your body's reaction to certain substances known as allergens that your body considers foreign invaders rather than the harmless substances they really are. When your body comes into contact with a specific allergen for the first time, it secretes a substance known as immunoglobulin E (IgE), an antibody specific to that allergen. IgE then attaches to the surface of specific cells in your body known as mast cells. These mast cells are found in large numbers in mucous membranes of your nose and in your skin, among others. They work to regulate inflammation by releasing various chemical compounds, including histamine.

After the first encounter with an allergen, future encounters cause a cascade of chemicals known as histamines, leukotrienes, and prostaglandins, which further triggers a range of allergic symptoms, including coughing, itchy eyes, nasal congestion, runny nose, sneezing, and sore throat.

The specific compound called histamine can even cause our airways to constrict, as in the case of allergy-induced asthma attacks, or cause blood vessels to become excessively permeable, causing fluid leakage or hives. Leukotrienes cause excessive secretion of mucus and the resulting signature symptoms of allergies: runny nose and increased mucus. Other substances known as prostaglandins can stimulate the release of histamine in the body, resulting in airway or tissue inflammation and a wide range of allergic symptoms.

The most common allergens include pollens, mold spores, dust, airborne contaminates, dust mites, pet dander, cockroaches, and environmental toxins, particularly those found in vehicle exhaust, cleaning products, personal-care products, and food additives. Every person is unique and, as a result, can have unique reactions to environmental substances. You can also develop a new allergy to something that was previously harmless. Alternatively, you can lose allergies just as quickly as they arrived, although that is uncommon unless you take certain measures to strengthen and balance your body's delicate immune and hormonal systems.

SYMPTOMS OF ALLERGIES

There are many allergy symptoms, but some of the most common include runny nose, nasal congestion, postnasal drip, itchy nose, itchy eyes, watering, tearing of the eyes, asthma, stuffy nose, cough, fatigue, weakness, sneezing, and sore throat. Allergies can also exacerbate other conditions, like asthma and sinus infections.

ASTHMA

Asthma is a serious respiratory condition that interferes with a person's ability to breathe. Typically asthmatics have some combination of bronchial muscle spasms, excess mucus production, and mucus lining swelling as a result of allergies, environmental irritants, infection, cold air, hormonal imbalances, exertion, and stress. The result is an asthma attack that can literally cause someone to suffocate if he or she doesn't get emergency medical intervention.

The incidence of asthma is on the rise. By some accounts, it has increased by more than 33 percent in just one decade, potentially the result of pollution, food additives, and excess inflammatory-causing meat, sugar, and fat consumption.

Some of the symptoms of asthma include wheezing, difficulty breathing, coughing, chest tightness, increased heart rate, sleep loss due to coughing and difficulty breathing, increased mucus flow, inflammation of the mucus linings of the lungs, and airway constriction in the bronchial muscles.

DIAGNOSING ALLERGIES

There are various types of tests for allergies. The most common medical ones include:

Blood testing for IgE antibodies. These blood tests show the specific substances to which your body had a full-blown allergic response involving IgE.

Allergy skin tests. Sometimes called *prick tests,* they involve a quick prick of the skin with a minute amount of a specific allergen to determine whether the skin will become inflamed and irritated. If it does, it means you have an allergy to this substance.

DO ALLERGY DRUGS SCARE YOU? THEY SHOULD!

There are several types of over-the-counter (OTC) and prescription medications used for treating allergy symptoms. These medications are classified as antihistamines, decongestants, a combination of antihistamine and decongestants, corticosteroids, and allergy shots.

Antihistamine Drugs

Antihistamine drugs block histamine receptors in the body, thereby reducing the symptoms of allergies. Released by part of the body's immune system known as mast cells, histamine is a naturally occurring substance in the body that causes blood vessels to dilate. In an allergic reaction, the immune system becomes hyperactive and overreacts to common, everyday substances such as pollens, molds, dust, animal dander, and so forth. When histamine is excessively released, it results in a runny nose, watery eyes, tissue swelling, and a constriction of the passageways of the lungs. Antihistamine drugs block receptors in the body so the histamine has less of an effect. Taken as eye drops, liquids, pills, and nasal sprays, antihistamines are largely OTC treatments used to diminish symptoms such as itchy eyes and nasal congestion. Although they can reduce symptoms, they do not address the causes of allergies.

Some of the most common antihistamine drugs include Allegra (fexofenadine), Benadryl (diphenhydramine), Zyrtec (cetirizine), and Claritin (loratadine); however, there are dozens of antihistamine drugs on the market.

> *Allegra (fexofenadine).* Fexofenadine is an antihistamine that is often used to treat sneezing, runny nose, itching, and watery eyes. The most common side effects include headaches, earaches, vomiting, back pain, body aches, chills,

coughing, diarrhea, dizziness, fevers, joint pain, muscle aches, nasal congestion, painful menstruation, runny or stuffy nose, sleepiness, sneezing, sore throat, and weakness.[2] You may notice that the drug can cause some of the same symptoms it is used to treat. You should not drive a vehicle or operate heavy machinery while using this drug, as it can cause drowsiness or dizziness and increase the risk of injury. Avoid alcohol while taking this medication. Fexofenadine should not be combined with the herb St. John's wort, as the herb increases blood levels of the drug. Conversely, ingestion of apple juice, grapefruit juice, or orange juice can decrease the blood levels of the drug, reducing its effectiveness.[3]

Benadryl (diphenhydramine). Also known by the names of Benylin, Tylenol Allergy Sinus, Tylenol Flu, Excedrin PM, and other brand names, diphenhydramine is primarily used to reduce the symptoms of sneezing, runny nose, itching, and watery eyes as well as to reduce swelling associated with allergic skin reactions. Although it is available on its own, it is also frequently combined with other drugs to address colds, flus, and other respiratory infections. Some of the side effects can include sedation, sleepiness, dizziness, loss of coordination, thickening of respiratory mucous secretions, depression, impaired motor skills, confusion, neck stiffness, difficulty swallowing, dementia, rash, eczema, nausea, tachycardia (quickening of the heart beat), heart palpitations, reduced blood pressure, anemia, and gastrointestinal (GI) upset.[4] You should not drive a vehicle or operate heavy machinery while using this drug, as it can cause drowsiness or dizziness and increase the risk of injury. Avoid alcohol while taking this medication, as it can significantly increase the drowsiness caused by the drug. This drug interacts with many other drugs, so you should consult your pharmacist if you're taking other medications. I'm unaware of any drug-herb interactions with diphenhydramine, but in theory, the drug may interact with the herb henbane (*Hyoscyamus niger*).[5] Because the herb can be toxic, it should only be used by a skilled herbalist, if at all, so it is not found in most herbal formulations.

Claritin (loratadine). Used to reduce the effects of histamine in the body, Claritin primarily reduces symptoms of sneezing, itching, watery eyes, runny nose, hives, or skin rashes. Some of the side effects can include headaches, fatigue, dry mouth, insomnia, nervousness, dizziness, abdominal pain, eye inflammation, flu-like symptoms, stomachache, earache, viral infection, impaired motor skills, and heart arrhythmias.[6] Because food can slow the absorption of the drug, it is usually recommended to take the drug on an empty stomach. Like other antihistamines, loratadine may cause drowsiness or dizziness. Avoid alcohol while taking this medication, as it can increase the drowsiness caused by the drug.[7]

Zyrtec (cetirizine). Like other antihistamines, cetirizine is used to alleviate the symptoms of sneezing, runny nose, itching, watery eyes, and hives. Some of the side effects of this drug can include drowsiness, fatigue, dry mouth, insomnia, headache, abdominal pain, irritability, nervousness, aggressive reactions, convulsions, nausea, vomiting, bronchitis, sinusitis, and asthma.[8] You may notice that the drug can cause some of the same symptoms it is used to treat. Avoid alcohol while taking this medication.[9]

Decongestants

Decongestant drugs do exactly what you'd expect based on the name: they reduce congestion in the nose and sinuses by constricting blood vessels in these areas. The vasoconstriction reduces swelling and inflammation in the nasal passages, thereby making it easier to breathe. They are taken either in pill form or by nasal sprays or drops to target the nasal and sinus region. Although there are other types of decongestants, most are known as pseudoephedrine. Pseudoephedrine is a synthetic, laboratory-derived version that is similar to the body's own hormone adrenaline, which is also known as epinephrine.[10] Ephedrine, which is available in prescription or nonprescription strengths, dilates the bronchi in the lungs, making it easier for asthmatics to breathe; pseudoephedrine is an OTC drug that has similar effects. Their brand names include Drixoral, Sudafed, Chlor-Trimeton, Suphedrin, and Suphedrine.

Some of the side effects of pseudoephedrine can include irregular or troubled heartbeat, shortness of breath, difficulty breathing, hallucinations, seizures, nervousness, restlessness, insomnia, headaches, increased sweating, weakness, trembling, nausea, vomiting, fast or pounding heartbeat, and difficult or painful urination.[11]

Both ephedrine and pseudoephedrine were originally derived from a plant known as ephedra, or by its scientific name, *Ephedra gerardiana*. The Chinese have been using this herb, which is known in Traditional Chinese Medicine (TCM) as Ma Huang, for thousands of years. The plant is a highly effective decongestant with far fewer side effects than the drug versions; however, it is not available in many places. Regulatory officials state diet pill abuses, many of which included ephedra, as the reason. Although some companies definitely abused this herb for profit and there were consumers who took far more than the recommended dosages, I suspect that ephedrine and pseudoephedrine sales are in the billion-dollar range, giving the pharmaceutical industry a significant reason to lobby regulators against ephedra. The herb provides stiff competition for these synthetic drugs and has far fewer side effects, giving Big Pharma cause for concern. Although it may be difficult to obtain, I'll share more information about the valuable allergy and decongestant herb ephedra in chapter 5.

Corticosteroids

Corticosteroids are a family of drugs that are synthetic derivatives of the adrenal gland hormones cortisone or cortisol made by the body. The adrenal glands are two triangular-shaped glands that sit atop the kidneys in the abdominal area. While the natural hormones are needed to sustain life, the synthetic drugs used in the treatment of asthma and some serious allergies have serious side effects, some of which include thrush (a yeast infection of the mouth), weakness, acne, weight gain, mood or behavioral changes, bone loss, slowing of growth, eye changes, headaches, nausea, vomiting, and insomnia.[12] They are available as inhalers to treat asthma, in topical forms to treat hives, or orally to address serious allergies. There are many names for corticosteroids, usually ending with the suffix -one, such as beclomethasone (brand names Beclovent, Beconase, Vanceril, Vancenase), fluticasone (brand names Flovent, Flonase), and triamcinolone (brand names Azmacort, Nasacort).

Allergy Shots/Immunotherapy

Allergy shots, or allergy vaccines or allergen immunotherapy as they are also known, are usually administered by vaccine once or twice a week. They are intended to desensitize the body to specific allergens. Each shot contains a minute amount of specific pollens, mold, dust, dander, bee venom, or other common allergen and is injected into the upper arm. Not only do they involve a significant time commitment to get a full course of treatment, but they can also be costly for those who do not have health care coverage for these treatments. Worse than that, they are painful and can cause serious reactions. This is particularly true for those people who tend to have life-threatening allergies, such as to bee venom. In some cases, allergy shots can cause the same allergic reactions they are used to treat. Allergy shots are intended to gradually increase your body's tolerance to allergens.

Some of the side effects of allergy shots include redness or swelling at the site of the vaccine, sneezing, nasal congestion, hives, throat swelling, wheezing, chest tightness, and anaphylactic shock; the latter is rare but a potentially life-threatening reaction to the vaccines used in allergy shots.[13]

MEDICATIONS: HIGH RISK, LOW REWARD

We might accept the serious side effects of many of these drugs if we knew they would cure us of what ails us, but the reality is that drugs don't cure diseases; they mitigate symptoms. And in most cases, they don't work much better, if at all better, than a placebo. According to Dr. Allen Roses, a scientist and the former global vice president of genetics at GlaxoSmithKline, "Most prescription medicines do not work on most people." He added, "The vast majority of drugs—more than 90 percent—only work on 30 to 50 percent of the people."[14]

Harvard University research found that approximately 50 percent of the effectiveness of pharmaceutical drugs can actually be linked to the placebo effect, not the actual effectiveness of the medication. Study participants were given either a pain drug or a placebo. When either the drug or placebo was administered with the message that it is an "effective treatment," both had significantly better results. When the real drug was switched with the placebo, the results were nearly the same, provided that the message of the effective treatment accompanied the pills.[15]

It should be fairly clear by now that the effectiveness of prescription drugs is much less than you may have believed. Much of their effectiveness can be attributed to the placebo effect or advertising or physician messaging that suggests that the drugs are effective. Additionally, when we refer to drugs as effective, we simply mean they reduce symptoms. Sadly, no drug has ever cured allergies. And considering the high cost, both financial and in terms of side effects, the minimal symptom improvement sometimes offered from pharmaceutical drugs is simply insufficient.

Consider a media release issued by the Orthomolecular Medicine News Service entitled "Does Anybody Still Believe Slam Pieces on Dietary Supplements?" In it, the organization reported that "the biological action of most prescription drugs can be duplicated with dietary supplements at far less cost and side effects. . . ."[16]

The nutrients, however, do not share the extensive list of side effects that accompany most prescription and OTC drugs, particularly in the category of pharmaceutically prepared analgesics. Twenty years ago, astute medical professionals who kept up on the research knew that nutrients could replace prescription drugs for treating disease.

As you'll soon discover in *Allergy-Proof Your Life*, foods, nutrients, natural medicines, and lifestyle modifications go a long way toward alleviating allergy symptoms and, in many cases I've personally witnessed, eliminating the allergies altogether.

Forget blaming bad genes for the conditions that ail you: allergies are included as pioneering research into a specific field known as nutrigenomics—the study of the effects of nutrition on the expression of DNA. Nutrigenomics has found that certain nutrients formed compounds that could actually "turn off" the expression of so-called bad genes.[17] While we once believed our genes were comparable to ticking time bombs just waiting to go off, leading scientists and nutritionists now know that what we eat and how we live plays a much greater role in preventing or even reversing the effects of our genes than we ever imagined possible.

If you believe drugs are the only effective options for allergies, think again. Besides that, many drugs actually cause the same symptoms they are taken to alleviate. The natural options I'll share with you over the coming chapters not only reduce allergy symptoms; they also strengthen and balance the body to quiet an overactive immune system and go to the root cause of the allergies themselves—which is *not* a drug deficiency disease as the pharmaceutical industry would have you believe.

2

Foods That Harm, Foods That Heal

WHEN I FIRST MET my husband, Curtis, he suffered from severe seasonal allergies. Sneezing, sniffling, itchy eyes, and nasal congestion seemed to be part of his springtime routine. We moved in together about six weeks after our first date. Yes, it was quick, but we were and still are madly in love and have been together for nearly nineteen years now.

When we embarked on our first joint grocery order, we decided to "divide and conquer": I picked up the fresh produce while Curtis tracked down the juice, pasta, and other staples. When he arrived back at the grocery cart, arms full of items on our list, I was shocked. I couldn't believe the junk he had gathered. From sugar-loaded cranberry juice to white pasta and freezer pastry dough, I hadn't expected so much junk from someone who was so fit and athletic. I said "that's not juice" after noticing the sugar-water-cranberry solution, and we had a good laugh about our different eating styles.

Already a holistic nutritionist with a focus on the use of food to heal disease for several years by the time Curtis and I had that first grocery shopping experience together, I quickly realized that my sweetheart's diet was playing a significant role in his allergy symptoms. I asked him if he would consider making dietary changes if they would likely help his seasonal allergies. Considering his love of the outdoors, as well as hiking, running, cycling, walking, he agreed.

I recommended eliminating all dairy products from his diet, including the ones hidden in his morning muffins and other baked goods that were a normal part of his diet. I also suggested that he significantly reduce all sugar from his diet for at least one month. My plan for Curtis involved eliminating all white-flour pastas and breads and any foods with trans fats and chemical food additives. I was impressed that he followed my plan to the letter for a full month. During that time, he observed that his allergies continuously improved and, by one month, were completely gone.

Curtis was pleasantly surprised that simply changing his diet reversed his seasonal allergies altogether. He also experienced more energy, increased vitality, better-quality sleep, and fewer headaches on this new eating plan. He stuck with the program most of the time but would occasionally enjoy a sugary treat. Curtis observed that if he ate too many of his old favorites, his allergy symptoms would come back, although they were never as severe as they once had been. And he felt empowered knowing that he could simply make dietary improvements and watch his seasonal allergies lift.

I have observed the dietary connection to seasonal allergies over and over again with many patients in my practice over the last twenty-five years. One eighteen-year-old young man exclaimed, "I can't believe that just by eliminating dairy products and sugar my allergies are gone!" Although it may seem hard to believe, my experience proves otherwise. And as you're about to learn, it is easier than you might think to eliminate these mucus-forming, allergy-aggravating foods from your diet. There are many excellent replacements for your favorite foods so you won't feel deprived. I eat some of the best food of my life, even though I don't eat dairy products and I rarely eat sweets made with sugar.

THE NOT-SO-SUGAR-COATED TRUTH ABOUT SUGAR

Sugar is not the safe addition to an otherwise healthy diet that manufacturers of sugary foods would have you believe. It is highly mucus forming and aggravates allergies. I put my clients on a minimum thirty-day low-sugar diet (and no, that doesn't mean adding artificial sweeteners), and as you learned from my husband's story, most of them see dramatic improvements in their environmental allergies even if they do nothing else and don't bother with supplements or herbs. Of course, if you want faster results, then I definitely recommend including other natural remedies, which I'll describe later in chapter 5.

In my experience, most asthma and allergy sufferers are sensitive to sugars of all kinds, natural or otherwise. It is best to cut back on all sweeteners and artificial sweeteners, the latter of which we'll discuss momentarily. Besides that, the average person eats far too much sugar, which depresses the immune system, throws off the delicate microbial balance in the intestines (more on this later), causes mucus to form, and can contribute to the nasal and sinus congestion of allergies. According to the US Department of Agriculture (USDA), the average person eats 156 pounds of added sugar every year. That doesn't include naturally present sugar in foods like fruit. Compare that with our ancestors' diet a century ago: they ate only about five pounds of sugar annually.

Soda is one of the worst sources of sugar, containing seven to eleven teaspoons per can, or the equivalent of thirty-nine milligrams of sugar per can, and much more than that for the supersized beverages now sold at many fast-food places. Sugar is insidious in our diet, hiding in many unsuspected places, including condiments, meat, french fries, and even in some salt—it's shocking but true.

Look for any ingredient that contains the suffix *-ose*, such as glucose, high-fructose corn syrup (HFCS), fructose, dextrose, maltose, and so forth. Even natural sweeteners like honey, pure maple syrup, agave nectar, and barley malt are high in sugars and should be used sparingly. Here are some of the surprising sources of hidden sugar identified by Nancy Appleton in her book *Lick the Sugar Habit*.

- The breading on most packaged and restaurant foods contains sugar.
- Hamburgers sold in restaurants often have corn syrup and dehydrated molasses added to reduce meat shrinkage during cooking.
- Before salmon is canned, it is often glazed with a sugar solution.
- Many meat packers feed sugar to animals prior to slaughter to "improve" the flavor and color of cured meat.
- Some fast-food restaurants sell poultry that has been injected with a sugar or honey solution.
- Some salt contains sugar! Seriously.
- Sugar is used in the processing of luncheon meats, bacon, and canned meats.
- Most bouillon cubes contain sugar (and usually monosodium glutamate [MSG] as well).
- Peanut butter tends to contain sugar.
- Dry cereals often contain high amounts of sugar.
- Almost half of the calories from commercial ketchup comes from sugar.
- More than 90 percent of the calories found in a can of cranberry sauce come from sugar.

This list is by no means complete. Sugar hides almost anywhere, and as it becomes increasingly genetically modified, it is important to reduce your consumption of it. Frequently, it is not even listed on food packages, making it doubly difficult to spot hidden sugar in the foods you eat. Additionally, it can take different forms. HFCS is one of the most prevalent forms of hidden sugar in packaged and prepared foods.

NINE REASONS TO AVOID HIGH-FRUCTOSE CORN SYRUP LIKE THE PLAGUE

If you take a look at most candy, cereal, bread, frozen food, yogurt, baby food, granola bars, salad dressing, crackers, condiments, or other processed food packages, you're sure to see HFCS on the ingredients list. It might even be easy to equate commonality with safety, assuming that that if HFCS really was damaging to your health, surely the Food and Drug Administration (FDA) would ban it, right? Wrong. Just because it has the name "corn" in it, which most people consider a healthy vegetable, combined with the fact that It is found almost everywhere doesn't make it safe to eat. But HFCS is one of the reasons our sugar consumption is so high.

The average American currently consumes fifty-five pounds of HFCS every year, which is a higher per capita consumption than any other country in the world.[1] If you're currently consuming HFCS–and most people are without even realizing it–it is likely contributing to your environmental allergies. But there are many reasons you might want to reconsider avoiding it like the plague:

Chronic Inflammation–HFCS perforates the gut lining, allowing partially digested food, fecal matter, and harmful bacteria to cross the intestinal wall directly into the blood. The result: inflammation and an overactive immune system caused by the body's own immune system attacks on these substances it perceives as foreign invaders. This overactive immune system and low-grade inflammation contributes to allergies and many other chronic illnesses. We'll discuss more about the gut-allergy connection in the next chapter.

Diabetes–Research at the University of Southern California and Oxford University found that HFCS is linked with diabetes, which may explain the rapidly growing rates of diabetes.[2] Their research, published in the medical journal *Global Public Health*, showed that HFCS consumption is linked to a 20 percent higher prevalence of diabetes in those who consume it over those who don't. They also determined that this higher incidence of diabetes occurred regardless of the total amount of sugar consumed or obesity levels.

Fatty Liver Disease–Consumption of HFCS has also been linked to fatty liver disease.[3] The sugary substance must be metabolized by the liver, and this puts a tremendous strain on this already hard-working organ.

Reproductive Disorders and *Cancer*–HFCS is largely made up of genetically modified corn because it is inexpensive to grow and has a high crop yield. But genetically modified foods have been linked in research to reproductive disorders[4] and cancer.[5]

Obesity–HFCS requires little to no digestion, so it is quickly absorbed into the bloodstream. As a result, the sugar causes rapid spikes in insulin production, which is the body's fat-storage hormone. Not only does your appetite increase, but your weight does as well. It's no surprise that high consumption of HFCS is linked to obesity.[6]

Energy Depletion–Sugar found in HFCS requires greater amounts of energy to be absorbed by the gut than other types of sugar. Each molecule requires two molecules of phosphorus, which it takes from our body's ATP. ATP is the body's energy currency, so you can probably imagine what happens over time when there are constant withdrawals and few deposits. Just like a bank account, you will become overdrawn. When this happens you experience energy depletion.[7]

Learning Impairment–Research also shows that the daily consumption of beverages sweetened with HFCS such as soda impaired learning and the ability to remember information, particularly when consumption occurs during adolescence.

Increased Blood Pressure and Heart Disease Risk–A study published in the *Journal of the American Society of Nephrology* found that even people who eat an otherwise healthy diet but consume HFCS are at risk of an increase in blood pressure by up to 32 percent. The study, conducted at the University of Colorado, found that the inflammation caused by HFCS leads to inflammation in the bloodstream, which causes the blood vessel walls to tighten, resulting in blood pressure increases.[8]

THE GOOD AND BAD OF SUGAR SUBSTITUTES

Before you panic thinking that you have to swear off all sweets, you'll be happy to know that there is an herb that works marvelously to replace sugar in many foods such as coffee, tea, and soda. Stevia, or *Stevia rebaudiana*, is a natural herb that tastes sweet but doesn't actually contain sugar molecules. As a result, it doesn't affect blood sugar levels or inflammation in the body and is therefore a healthy option for a healthy body. It is naturally between three hundred and one thousand times sweeter than sugar, depending whether you're using the whole herb or the liquid extract. I personally find that liquid stevia has the best taste and least aftertaste, but I have found powdered ones that are excellent as well.

Make the switch from sugar to the naturally sweet herb stevia, which is available in many forms, including liquid extract, powdered extract, or powdered herb. Be aware that some manufacturers of the powdered extract of stevia include other sweeteners alongside the herb, so these products are best avoided.

Because stevia is naturally sweet, you won't need much to sweeten your tea, coffee, or other foods and beverages. Just a few drops sweetens coffee or tea. The powder usually comes with what looks like a doll-sized spoon because that's all you'll need for most beverages.

Baking with stevia poses some challenges because, other than sweetening, it doesn't have the same chemical properties of sugar, such as caramelizing when heated or becoming chewy in cookies. Also, because you use so little stevia, it may throw off the traditional dry to wet ingredient ratio if you try to substitute stevia. So you may need to experiment a bit with your recipes, or you can try some of the delicious options that I created in the last chapter of this book.

If you have a sweet tooth, opt for a piece of fruit or sweeten your beverages or foods with natural stevia (avoid products with maltodextrin or other added sweeteners).

If you're thinking that aspartame or another artificial sweetener is a better option than sugar, think again. Artificial sweeteners may have fewer calories than the real thing, but they are anything but healthy and have no place in a health-supporting diet. They're not just bad for you; they're linked to many serious illnesses and should never have been allowed in our food supply.

Only one year after aspartame was approved by the FDA, its own task force learned that some of the original data showcasing aspartame's safety had been falsified to hide results showing that animals fed aspartame had developed seizures and brain tumors.[9] The artificial sweetener was never recalled. Aspartame has also been linked to the formation of various types of cancer, including brain cancer. There is also a 43 percent increased risk of experiencing a stroke or heart attack when a person drinks more than one diet soda daily.

According to the authors of the book *The Hundred-Year Lie*, when a diet drink containing aspartame is stored at 85 degrees Fahrenheit for a week or longer, "There is no aspartame left in the soft drinks, just the components it breaks down into, like formaldehyde, formic acid, and diketopiperazine, a chemical which can cause brain tumors. All of these substances are known to be toxic to humans."[10] Combine these ingredients with a leaky gut, which you'll learn more about later in this book, and you have a recipe for inflammation in the body. That's because these chemicals can hijack the body's normal process for absorbing nutrients through the lining of the gut, but when the gut lining is damaged, as is often the case in allergy sufferers, then these toxic chemicals can gain direct access to the bloodstream, where they can cause further damage and inflammation—another underlying factor for allergies.

Allergies are just the start of how aspartame is damaging to the body. Ironically, considering its name and reputation as a "diet" drink, drinking diet soda is more likely to make a person overweight or obese. It is linked to a 34 percent increase of metabolic syndrome, along with its telling symptoms of high cholesterol and abdominal obesity.[11] Just two cans of diet soda daily have been linked to a 500 percent increase in waist size.[12] By skipping aspartame, you're likely to lose weight if you're overweight. And because a Harvard University study found that drinking diet soda daily doubles a person's risk of kidney disease, by eliminating this beverage you'll have a reduced incidence of kidney disease as well.[13] You'll even maintain stronger teeth, as diet soda is extremely acidic and has been linked to dental enamel erosion.[14]

Aspartame isn't the only artificial sweetener that poses a threat to health. Saccharin and sucralose should be avoided as well.

Saccharin, also known as Sweet'N Low, Sweet Twin, and Necta Sweet, is touted as a safe sugar substitute, but it is actually a coal tar derivative. When it was first researched to cause bladder tumors in rats, it was still allowed to stay in the marketplace due to consumer demand as long as it carried a warning label that it may be harmful to health. Experts still consider saccharin a "probable carcinogen"[15] that also causes breathing difficulties, headaches, skin conditions, and diarrhea in some people.

Sucralose, or Splenda, is not a good option either. Although it is widely touted as a natural sweetener, it was created in a laboratory by altering sugar molecules in a way that could not appear in nature. It was barely tested before being launched with massive marketing campaigns as a supposedly healthy alternative to sugar. According to research by Dr. Joseph Mercola, the FDA only conducted two human studies on sucralose prior to its approval for use in food. The longest study lasted a mere four days and exclusively examined sucralose for its effects on tooth decay, not any other health effects. Additionally, when sucralose was tested to determine its absorption in the body, only eight men were studied.

Besides insufficient or skewed testing, sucralose is simply not the natural sweetener the manufacturer claims it is. It may start as a sugar molecule, but that's the end of the similarities between sugar and sucralose. Three chlorine molecules are added to each sugar molecule, which, according to Dr. Mercola, means sucralose "has been altered to the point that it's actually closer to DDT and Agent Orange than sugar."[16]

Sucralose has been linked with many serious conditions, including the following:

- allergic reactions such as facial swelling and swelling of the eyelids, tongue, throat, or lips
- allergic skin reactions such as itching, swelling, redness, weeping, crusting, rashes, eruptions, or hives
- anxiety
- blood sugar increases
- blurred vision
- breathing problems, including shortness of breath, coughing, chest tightness, and wheezing
- depression
- dizziness
- gastrointestinal complaints, including diarrhea, vomiting, nausea, bloating, gas, or pain
- headaches
- heart palpitations
- itchy, swollen, watery, or bloodshot eyes
- joint pains

- mental fog
- migraines
- seizures
- sinus congestion, runny nose, or sneezing
- weight gain

You'll notice that many of the symptoms actually mimic environmental allergy symptoms. It's essential to eliminate this artificial sweetener and other artificial ingredients from your diet to restore your immune system health and eliminate allergies.

OTHER ADDITIVES TO SUBTRACT FROM YOUR DIET

There are hundreds of additives in packaged, processed, and prepared foods—what I call the Three Ps. Many of these additives put a strain on the body and actually contribute to low-grade inflammation and other conditions linked to allergies. Some of the worst culprits include monosodium glutamate (MSG) and carrageenan.

MSG is linked to inflammation, hormonal imbalances, headaches, and many other symptoms. It is almost always found in processed, prepared, and packaged foods, including soups, spice mixtures, infant formulas, soy "meat" products, baby foods, bottled sauces, salad dressings, croutons, protein powders, and vaccines. Sadly, it is rarely listed as MSG or monosodium glutamate on the labels of foods. Instead, it appears in the guise of the following:

- hydrolyzed vegetable protein
- hydrolyzed protein
- hydrolyzed plant protein
- plant protein extract
- sodium caseinate

- calcium caseinate
- yeast extract
- textured vegetable protein
- autolyzed yeast
- hydrolyzed oat flour

Additionally, it frequently appears in the form of flavoring, natural flavoring, seasoning, or spices on the labels of food. Because it can be difficult to remember the myriad disguises of MSG, I tell my clients to avoid foods that include the following terms in the list of ingredients: *hydrolyzed, isolate, caseinate,* spices/seasonings, or flavors (natural or artificial).

You should also avoid the food additive known as carrageenan. It's an additive that is so ubiquitous in the food industry that it is even found in most packaged foods and restaurant sauces, and even many foods that have been labeled "certified organic" contain the questionable ingredient. Although the additive starts out harmless enough (it comes from the seaweed known as Irish moss), it is then processed to extract the ingredient known as carrageenan, which acts as a thickener or emulsifier for many prepared foods. Once this ingredient has been extracted, it turns from an otherwise healthy food to one that causes widespread inflammation in the body.

Like most people, I originally thought that carrageenan was a harmless extract from seaweed, so I didn't give it much consideration. Then while conducting my regular health and nutrition research, I read that scientists were giving animals carrageenan to induce inflammation as a way to prepare them for scientific studies exploring anti-inflammatory drugs. That was the first I'd heard of carrageenan being used in this way. So I began to investigate.

Dr. Joanne Tobacman has conducted many studies on the effects of carrageenan consumption, including a recent one in the *Journal of Diabetes Research*.[17] After eating carrageenan for only six days, animals fed carrageenan developed glucose intolerance, which is an umbrella term used to describe impaired metabolism involving excessively high blood sugar levels. Dr. Tobacman found that the food additive caused blood sugar levels to skyrocket and indicates that it may lead to the development of diabetes. She indicates that because carrageenan used in animals' diets commonly causes diabetes, the additive could be used for mouse models of the study of diabetes.

She also found that carrageenan causes intestinal and systemic inflammation in animal studies.[18] Considering that inflammation is a well-established factor in most chronic diseases, including heart disease, diabetes, cancer, arthritis, pain disorders, and many others, any food additive in common use is a serious concern. Dr. Tobacman also indicates that the amount of carrageenan found in most peoples' diets is sufficient to cause inflammation.[19]

Carrageenan is found in common foods, including infant formula, ice cream, cream, butter, soy milk, almond milk, rice milk, cottage cheese, sour cream, yogurt, coffee creamer, vegan cheese alternatives, egg nog, protein supplements, aloe vera gel, deli meat, juice, pudding, pizza, chocolate bars, coffee beverages, and many other packaged foods. Additionally, some supplements, particularly those involving gel caps, commonly contain carrageenan. And most grocery store rotisserie chickens typically contain the additive. Even many organic and certified organic foods contain carrageenan. To find out if the organic foods you use contain carrageenan that might not be listed on the label, check out the "Shopping Guide to Avoiding Organic Foods with Carrageenan" list compiled by the Cornucopia Institute at www .cornucopia.org.

In addition to MSG and carrageenan, be sure to avoid food containing artificial colors and preservatives. The preservatives known as sodium benzoate and potassium benzoate, once ingested, form a toxic chemical known as benzene in the presence of vitamin C. According to an interview with Peter Piper, a professor of molecular biology and biotechnology at the University of Sheffield in the United Kingdom, "These chemicals have the ability to cause severe damage to DNA in the mitochondria to the point that they totally inactivate it—they knock it out altogether." Additionally, these preservatives have been linked to allergic conditions like hives and asthma, according to the Center for Science in the Public Interest.[20]

THE DAIRY DILEMMA

Forget what dairy marketing bureaus would have you believe—dairy is not the health food it has been touted as. When it comes to seasonal and environmental allergies, I have found that dairy products are one of the worst culprits. It may seem like an unusual connection, but I have observed the disappearance of allergies in countless clients over the past twenty-five years when they follow a dairy-free and low-sugar diet plan. For most people, these two simple dietary changes are sufficient to eliminate seasonal allergies as long as this type of diet is followed. Let's explore some of the problems with dairy products.

Dairy products are highly mucus forming and can contribute to a whole host of respiratory conditions, including nasal and sinus congestion as well as lung troubles like asthma. Milk and other dairy products tend to be difficult to digest. Baby cows that drink their mother's milk have four times the stomach capacity as humans, but most humans struggle with the digestion of dairy products. Most people assume that only those who have symptoms of lactose intolerance have difficulty digesting dairy products, but there are many other symptoms linked to their digestion, including indigestion, heartburn, abdominal cramps, aching joints, sinus troubles, nasal congestion, arthritis, and many others.

As if cow's milk wasn't hard enough to digest, most milk is homogenized, which denatures the milk's proteins, making it even harder to digest. Many peoples' bodies react to these proteins as though they are "foreign invaders" causing their immune systems to overreact. Research also links homogenized milk to heart disease. Additionally, during this homogenization process all the enzymes that help digest milk are destroyed. Further, any beneficial bacteria that would have predigested the milk products, making them easier for us to digest, are also killed.

But difficulty digesting proteins isn't the only issue. Due to our commercialization processes involved in the growth of dairy cows, many foreign substances find their way into the cows and are then passed along to the milk they produce, which ultimately end up in our bodies when we drink or eat products made with milk. Pesticides in cow feed find their way into milk and dairy products that we consume. Not only are the naturally present hormones in cow's milk stronger than human hormones, throwing off our delicate hormone balance, but the animals are routinely given synthetic hormones to plump them up and increase milk production. These hormones further throw off our hormonal balance.

As soon as I tell people to stop eating dairy products, they inevitably ask me, "But how will I get my calcium?" We have been duped into thinking that dairy products equal calcium in the same way we think meat equals protein. Although dairy products are undoubtedly high in calcium, dairy products are difficult to digest, which means that we actually absorb very little of the calcium found in these products. The calcium found in plant-based foods is far superior to dairy products because it is much easier to digest and absorb.

Before you panic about increasing your risk of osteoporosis if you give up dairy products, you might be surprised to learn that research shows that the countries whose citizens consume the most dairy products have the *highest* incidence of osteoporosis, with Americans and Canadians having some of the highest rates of the disease. Some of the foods that have high amounts of highly absorbable calcium include almonds, almond butter, broccoli, carrot juice, carrots, dark leafy greens, kale, kelp, navy beans, oats, sesame seeds, sesame butter (tahini), soymilk and tofu (organic only, as soy is heavily contaminated by genetically modified organisms, or GMOs), wild salmon, and sardines.

Replace dairy products like milk, cream, butter, ice cream, and cheese with dairy-free beverages like almond or coconut milk or cashew or coconut cream, coconut butter or a vegan butter substitute instead of butter, and cashew- or coconut-based ice creams. Additionally, there are many excellent dairy-free cheeses now on the market. Avoid ones with casein, which is a dairy product derivative that is mucus forming and difficult to digest. Many of today's vegan cheeses are delicious, artisanal options that are far from the original ones that hit the market decades ago. So if you haven't tried them lately, you might want to explore dairy-free cheeses. Also, there are a wide variety of styles and tastes, so if you don't like one, try a different variety.

BEYOND THE MEAT MYTH

Most foods contain protein, including fruits and vegetables, yet many people still believe the myth that meat is the best or only source of protein. This myth and the dietary habits that support it are having serious health ramifications.

The average person in the United States or Canada eats more than 248 pounds of meat every year. That's about the equivalent of eating a whole pig each year and comprises about 40 percent of the typical person's diet. Most health and nutrition experts agree that meat should not exceed 10 percent of our overall food intake, but most people eat four times that amount. When you consider that our ancestors ate an estimated 5 percent of their total food intake in the form of meat and that they ate substantially less food than us, you might begin to understand why this extremely high amount of meat consumption is a problem. Yet people still ask me, "If I cut back on meat, where will I get my protein?" The food pyramids and other equally irrelevant systems of nutrition we were taught in school have led us to believe that we will be protein starved if we don't eat the whopping amounts of meat we consume daily.

Sorry, meat lovers, but a study at the University of Columbia found that eating bacon fourteen times a month was linked to damaged lung function and an increased risk of respiratory diseases.[21] Eating processed foods like bacon also increases the risk of dying young.[22] And according to research in the journal *Circulation*, daily consumption of processed meats like bacon, sausage, and deli meats can increase the risk of heart disease by 42 percent and diabetes by 19 percent.[23] Although some meat is fine, processed meat is not part of a health-building, immune system–restoring diet and is best avoided.

High-protein diets like Atkins and South Beach have left many people thinking that animal products are the only foods that contain protein. That is simply not true: fruits, vegetables, nuts, seeds, legumes, and whole grains all contain protein. Most people actually eat excessive amounts of protein from animal sources, which requires a tremendous amount of energy for digestion. Additionally, excessive meat—and, incidentally, dairy—consumption is linked to imbalanced levels of certain microorganisms in the gut, according to Harvard University research published in the journal *Nature*.[24]

It has long been known that diet influences the type and activity of the trillion microorganisms residing in the human gut, but Harvard scientists found that even what we eat in the short term can have drastic effects on the type and numbers of microbes in our gut and their capacity to increase inflammation in the GI tract, which can cause inflammation anywhere in the body, including the sinuses, lungs, and nasal passageways. Additionally, this GI inflammation can also result in immune system imbalances like the overreactivity of the immune system to dust, pollens, molds, or other environmental substances. I'll share more about this GI-immune system link in the next chapter.

The Harvard scientists discovered that microbes found in the food, including bacteria, fungi, and viruses, quickly colonize the gut. They also found that an animal-based diet such as the SAD caused the growth of microorganisms that are capable of triggering inflammatory bowel disease within only two days of eating these foods. Other research links inflammation-causing microbes to the degradation of our health, suggesting that the Harvard study has potentially far-reaching implications for the prevention and treatment of many conditions, allergies included.

The scientists put volunteers on a meat and cheese diet, then switched them to a fiber-rich, plant-based diet to track the effect on intestinal microbes. The study participants ate a breakfast of eggs and bacon, a lunch of ribs and briskets, and then salami, prosciutto, and assorted cheeses for dinner, along with pork rind snacks. After a break from eating this diet, the volunteers ate a plant-based diet of granola for breakfast; jasmine rice, cooked onions, tomatoes, squash, garlic, peas, and lentils for lunch; and a similar dinner, with bananas and mangoes for snacks.

The scientists analyzed the volunteers' microbes before, during, and after each meal. The effects of the meat and cheese were almost immediate. The abundance of bacteria shifted about a day after the food hit the gut. After three days on either diet, the bacteria in the gut also changed their behavior.

Lead scientist Lawrence David, PhD, admits that the meat-and-cheese diet used in his experiments was extreme; however, such an extreme diet helps paint a clear picture of the outcome of a diet heavy in meat and cheese—and frankly, this is a typical diet for many people who use high-protein diets or follow the SAD. This high-animal-protein diet clearly demonstrates the microbial impact of animal-protein-rich diets. Dr. David said in an interview with the online journal *NPR*, "I love meat . . .

but I will say that I definitely feel a lot more guilty ordering a hamburger . . . since doing this work."

If you want to restore your health and address the inflammation and immune system overreactions involved in allergies, you'll want to reconsider reaching for that bacon-wrapped sausage, cheese platter, or burger. Does that mean you have to become a vegan? Of course not—unless you want to. It means that you should cut back on meat as your source of protein and move to an increasingly plant-based diet.

Before you panic wondering where you will get your protein, here are some of the best nonmeat sources of protein:

- avocado
- coconut
- legumes, such as kidney beans, black beans, navy beans, pinto beans, Romano beans, chickpeas, soybeans, and edamame (green soybeans)
- nuts (preferably raw, unsalted), including almonds, Brazil nuts, cashews, macadamia nuts, pecans, pistachios, and walnuts
- quinoa
- seeds, such as chia seeds, flaxseeds, hemp seeds, pumpkin seeds, sunflower seeds, and sesame seeds
- soy products (organic only, as soy is heavily genetically modified), such as tofu, miso, and tempeh
- dairy alternatives, including almond milk, coconut milk, hemp seed milk, and soy milk

You may notice that protein powders are not on the list. That's because many are heavily processed, sugar laden, or contain neurotoxic MSG in one of its many guises, particularly protein "isolates." Ground seeds, like those mentioned on the list, are a much better way to add protein to your smoothies than by using protein powders.

A GRAIN OF TRUTH

It's important to select the right types of carbohydrates, or carbs, to include in your diet to help reset your immune system to reduce or eliminate allergies. Some of the carbs to avoid include white potatoes, white rice, and white flour and foods made with it. These foods act similarly to sugar in the body, causing wild blood sugar fluctuations and the resulting inflammation and changes to the gut terrain. Some of these bad carb foods include pastries, doughnuts, candies, cakes, white bread, "multigrain" bread (which is actually mostly white flour with a handful of grains added to it), and whole-wheat bread (which also tends to be largely white flour with a small amount of whole wheat added to it). Whole wheat has been heavily sprayed with harmful inflammation-causing pesticides and is best avoided. That doesn't mean you have to give up all your favorite foods. Most bread, cakes, pastries and other foods can be made with whole-grain flour that does not have the same inflammatory effect on your body. Here are some suggestions about which grains to enjoy and which to avoid:

Enjoy This	Avoid That
100 percent whole-grain bread (no wheat)	white bread, whole-wheat bread
brown rice pasta	white wheat pasta, semolina pasta
brown rice vermicelli	white rice vermicelli, egg noodles
brown rice, brown basmati rice, black rice	white rice, basmati rice, rice blends
quinoa	couscous
sweet potatoes or Jerusalem artichokes	white, yellow, or red potatoes

Many whole grains such as buckwheat, millet, oats, quinoa, or wild rice can be made into gourmet whole-grain dishes with chopped vegetables and spices, or they can be cooked and made into hearty salads with the addition of chopped fruits, vegetables, and seasonings.

IS GLUTEN AGGRAVATING YOUR ASTHMA?

Many asthma sufferers are sensitive to gluten, which is found in wheat, rye, oats, barley, and many other grains and products containing them. Many baking powders, soy sauces, artificial food colors, emulsifiers, and other ingredients found in convenience food also contain gluten. Some great gluten-free options include quinoa, millet, buckwheat (yes, the name can be confusing, but there is no gluten in buckwheat), coconut flour, brown rice, black rice, red rice, and wild rice. If you suffer from allergy-induced asthma, it is best to avoid gluten.

WHOLE GRAINS TO ADD TO YOUR DIET

Whole grains have gotten a bad rap in recent years. The average person eats refined grain products like white flour and white rice and avoids whole grains like the plague. Meanwhile low-carb dieters swear off whole grains in favor of high-protein options like meat and poultry under false pretenses that all grains are evil. Whole grains help stabilize blood sugar, are precursors to essential brain hormones, boost mood, and help keep us regular.

There are many delicious and highly nutritious whole grains to choose from, so adding whole grains to your allergy-eliminating diet needn't be daunting. Although there are many options, here are seven whole grains to get you started: barley, brown rice, kamut (pronounced *ka-MOOT*), spelt, oats, quinoa (pronounced *KEEN-wah*), and wild rice.

Barley

Used as far back as the Stone Age for currency, food, and med-icine, barley is a great addition to a healthy diet. Because barley contains plentiful amounts of both soluble and insoluble fiber, it helps aid bowel regularity. It contains ninety-six calories, twenty-two grams of carbohydrates, and three grams of fiber per half cup of cooked barley. Unrefined barley contains abun-dant amounts of potassium and also has lots of magnesium, manganese, vitamin E, B-complex vitamins, zinc, copper, iron, calcium, protein, sulfur, and phosphorus. This versatile ingredi-ent can be added to soups, stews, cereal, salads, pilaf, or ground into flour for baked goods or desserts. Barley contains gluten and should be avoided if you suspect you have gluten sensitivity.

Brown Rice

Brown rice is more nutritious and a much better option than white rice. Unlike white rice, it offers you vitamin E (import-ant for healthy immunity, skin, and many essential functions in your body) and is high in fiber. White rice is stripped of its fiber and most nutrients too. In its whole brown rice form, it con-tains high amounts of the minerals manganese, magnesium, and selenium. It also contains tryptophan, which helps with sleep. Brown rice can easily replace white rice in almost any recipe—soups, stews, and as a base for curries.

Buckwheat

Unrelated to wheat, buckwheat is actually not a grain at all but rather the seed of a plant related to rhubarb. As is often the case with seeds, buckwheat's nutritional value surpasses grains. It is low on the glycemic index, preventing rapid spikes in blood sugar that cause inflammation, mood swings, and weight gain. Buckwheat has more protein than corn, millet, rice, or wheat and is high in the amino acids lysine and arginine, both of which tend to be deficient in grains and are essential for a healthy heart and strong immunity to illness. It is naturally gluten-free, making it an excellent option for celiacs, those with gluten allergies, or anyone trying to avoid gluten. Because of its amino acid content, it can boost the protein content of beans and grains eaten in the same day. Buckwheat is unsurpassed in its ability to normalize cholesterol levels.

In addition to being low glycemic, its protein and fiber content help normalize blood sugar levels. Research published in the *Journal of Agricultural and Food Chemistry* showed that a single dose of buckwheat seed extract lowered high blood glucose levels by 12 to 19 percent within 90 to 120 minutes. Buckwheat has been shown to work in the same way as hypertension drugs, reducing levels of angiotensin converting enzyme (ACE), reducing hypertension without the nasty drug side effects. It is also a good source of tryptophan, which helps ensure a sound night's sleep. It is high in rutin, a natural flavonoid that helps extend the activity of vitamin C and other antioxidant nutrients. One cup of cooked buckwheat contains about eighty-six milligrams of magnesium—which boosts heart and muscle health and is necessary for the proper functioning of hundreds of enzymes in the body and, therefore, hundreds of processes. A study published in the *Journal of Gastroenterology* showed that a diet high in insoluble fiber like that found in buckwheat can help women avoid gallstones. The study was conducted on women, but the results are likely the same for men. One cup of cooked buckwheat contains almost 20 percent of your required daily intake of fiber. Diets high in fiber have been shown to significantly reduce the risk of colon cancer.

Use buckwheat flour along with your flour of choice to make pancakes, bread, muffins, and other baked goods. A traditional preparation of kasha (roasted whole buckwheat) is prepared in a stock of onions, parsley, and olive oil. Cook on its own or with equal parts of oats (gluten-free oats if you want a gluten-free breakfast), and top with berries as a hot breakfast cereal. Add cooked buckwheat to soups or stews to add flavor and nutrition. It cooks in under twenty minutes, making it a much healthier alternative than white rice and much faster than most whole grains.

Kamut and Spelt

Kamut and spelt are ancient grains that are part of the wheat family. Sometimes people with wheat allergies can tolerate kamut or spelt. Both of these tasty grains have higher nutritional value than whole wheat. Spelt is packed with the minerals manganese, magnesium, and copper and also contains high amounts of the mood-regulating and energy-boosting B-vitamins niacin, thiamine, and riboflavin. Choose kamut or spelt bread or pasta to replace white options. Kamut and spelt contain gluten and should be avoided if you suspect you have gluten sensitivity.

Oats

Oats are good for your body in many ways. They help stabilize blood sugar and lower cholesterol, and they are high in protein and fiber. Oats are available in many forms, including instant, steel-cut, rolled, bran, groats, flakes, and flour. The best options are the less refined ones like steel-cut, rolled, flakes, and bran. Oat flour is an excellent substitute for wheat flour in baking recipes. A good source of minerals like manganese, selenium, magnesium, and the sleep aid tryptophan, oats have been shown in many studies to also assist with lowering cholesterol and reducing the risk of heart disease. Although oats are naturally gluten-free, be sure to choose certified gluten-free oats if you are sensitive to gluten.

Quinoa

Quinoa, a staple of the ancient Incas who revered it as sacred, is not a true grain but rather seed. Surprisingly, it is related to spinach and Swiss chard. If you're not already enjoying this delicious food, there are many reasons to start. Because quinoa does not contain gluten, it is a good choice for anyone suffering from allergies. Unlike wheat, which is mucus forming, quinoa does not have the same mucus-forming properties. What's more, most grains lack one or more of the essential amino acids, making them incomplete. But quinoa packs an amino acid punch: it is a complete protein and is rich in nutrients, including manganese, iron, magnesium, B-vitamins, and fiber. In studies, quinoa is a proven aid for migraine sufferers, likely due to its magnesium and riboflavin content. Magnesium helps relax muscles, and riboflavin helps reduce the frequency of migraine attacks and improves energy metabolism within brain and muscle cells; this is valuable if your allergies are linked to migraines or headaches. And like most whole grains, it lessens the risk for heart disease. Quinoa also contains the building blocks for superoxide dismutase—an important antioxidant that helps protect the energy centers of your cells from free-radical damage. This enzyme also helps reduce the risk of free-radical damage linked to allergies. As if that weren't enough reasons to love this tiny seed, quinoa lessens the risk for heart disease and helps with heart arrhythmias.

Wild Rice

Not a true grain, wild rice is actually a type of aquatic grass seed that is native to the United States and Canada. It tends to be a bit pricier than other grains, but its high protein content and nutty flavor make wild rice worth every penny. It's an excellent choice for people with celiac disease or those who have gluten or wheat sensitivities. At eighty-three calories per half cup of cooked rice, it also has a lower caloric content than many grains. And wild rice is high in fiber. Add it to soups, stews, salads, and pilaf. It's important to note that wild rice is black. There are many blends of white and wild rice, which primarily consist of refined white rice. Be sure to use only real wild rice, not the blends.

COOKING GUIDE FOR WHOLE GRAINS

The following water amounts and cooking times are based on one cup of grain. As for all whole grains, add water and grain in a pot and bring to a boil. Once boiling, reduce to low heat to simmer for the amount of cooking time specified.

Barley (pearled): three cups water, fifteen minutes cooking time

Brown rice: two cups water, forty-five minutes cooking time

Buckwheat: one-and-a-half cups water, twenty minutes cooking time

Oats (quick cooking): two to three cups water, twelve to twenty minutes cooking time

Oats (rolled): two to three cups water, forty to fifty minutes cooking time

Quinoa: two cups water, fifteen minutes cooking time

Wild rice: three cups water, fifty to sixty minutes cooking time

Kamut and spelt can be cooked as whole grains but are most commonly used as whole-grain flour in breads and other baked goods.

FATS: THE GOOD, THE BAD, AND THE UGLY

Most packaged, processed, prepared, or fast foods actually contain unhealthy fats from margarine, lard or shortening, or rancid oils or from the processes in which they are prepared, such as frying or cooking at excessively high temperatures. These harmful fats contribute to inflammation in the body.

The typical diet, if it contains any healthy essential fatty acids, usually includes fats from meat and poultry or from nuts and seeds. Most diets are high in essential fatty acids known as omega-6s. Omega-6 fatty acids are found in the highest concentrations in corn, sunflower, and safflower oils, as well as in the meat of animals that eat a diet high in these fats. Although these fats are healthy in a ratio of one-to-one or even two-to-one of omega-6s to omega-3s (another essential fatty acid that the body must get from food), most people eat a twenty-to-one ratio. This excess worsens and even causes inflammation in the body. Eating too many omega-6 fatty acids in contrast to omega-3 fatty acids will produce substances in the body that will trigger or worsen existing inflammation. Yet that is exactly what the SAD contains: too many omega-6s and not enough omega-3 fatty acids.

Consuming oils like corn oil, safflower oil, sunflower oil, or "vegetable oil," which is usually a combination of corn, canola, and/or safflower oil, along with eating the meat of animals fed these fats in their diets, can worsen inflammation in the body, aggravate allergies, and negate the beneficial effects of healthy oils. Although many people know that fish (not the battered and fried variety) can be a healthier food choice thanks to its omega-3 fatty acid content, few people realize that if you eat a salad in which the dressing is made with one of the above-mentioned oils along with a piece of fatty fish, the oil in the salad will undo the benefits of eating the fish. Another example is tuna fish or sardines made into tuna salad or served on a sandwich alongside mayonnaise. The mayonnaise and the oils in the bread will counter any positive effects of eating the fish and aggravate low-grade inflammation in the body that leads to a wide range of possible health problems, including allergies and asthma.

Also, be sure to avoid peanuts, peanut oil, and foods cooked in peanut oil, as they tend to contain many aflatoxins (mold-like substances), which aggravate allergies, asthma, and inflammation.

Fishing for the Truth

There are many foods that are scientifically proven, all-natural anti-inflammatories. The most popular are foods that contain omega-3 fatty acids. Omega-3s are found in fatty cold-water fish like salmon, mackerel, sardines, anchovies, and tuna. Omega-3s convert in the body into hormone-like substances that decrease inflammation in the gut and throughout the whole body, reducing the likelihood or effects of immune system imbalances. Eating fish oil or supplementing with fish oil capsules daily can go a long way toward restoring your immune system health and reducing inflammation.

More Sources of Beneficial Omega-3s

Other foods with high amounts of omega-3 fatty acids include flaxseeds and flaxseed oil, walnut oil and raw walnuts, and dark leafy greens like spinach and kale. Do not heat or cook with flaxseed oil; it is best reserved for salad dressings or as a topping for steamed vegetables or baked potatoes. Walnut oil, although a bit pricy, is an excellent cooking oil or base for salad dressings and a great way to add more omega-3 fatty oils to your diet.

Where There's Smoke, There's Fire

It's not just the misplaced ratio of essential fatty acids that predisposes us to inflammation; it is also the quality of the oils we eat. All oils have different smoke points—the temperature above which the oil begins to smoke and is no longer healthy to eat. When oils smoke, their delicate essential oils become damaged, causing inflammation and, in some cases, also becoming carcinogenic. Because of this, oils that have extremely low smoke points, such as flaxseed oil, should never be heated. Olive oil smokes at about 320°F, whereas macadamia nut oil reaches its smoke point around 413°F. Like olive oil, walnut oil has a smoke point of about 320°F and should therefore be used on low to medium heat. Most oils sold in grocery stores, however, have been heated to extremely high temperatures during their processing and packaging, even before you get them home and begin to cook with them. These overheated or rancid oils no longer support joint health and actually create inflammation in the body. Extra virgin olive oil is the exception. Some grocery stores are moving to refrigerated, cold-pressed virgin oils, but this is still fairly rare. Most health food stores offer healthier, refrigerated, cold-pressed oils.

The Fried and True

I probably don't need to explain that fried foods such as french fries, onion rings, potato chips, and nachos cause inflammation. Most people know these items are not healthy choices and have no redeeming health quality. That's because the oils used in frying are frequently heated to excessive temperatures, often before they are even bottled for cooking and then again during the frying process. The oils are then used over and over again. When these oils are heated past their smoke point or are reused regularly, they become inflammation-causing oils. What you might not realize, however, is that these foods contribute to inflammation and need to be eliminated from your diet.

SEVEN MYTHS ABOUT OMEGA FATTY ACIDS

Considering all the talk of omega-3, -6, -7, and -9 fatty acids, you may be left a bit confused as to which ones you should be eating and which to avoid. To help you decipher the truth from the myth, here are the seven most common myths about omega fatty acids.

Myth #1: All omega fatty acids are equal. **Fact**: There is a big difference between the different types of omega fatty acids. Omega-3 fatty acids are anti-inflammatory, for example, whereas omega-6s are pro-inflammatory.

Myth #2: You should eat as many omega fatty acids as possible. **Fact**: Because most people already get excessive amounts of omega-6s, you should cut down on omega-6s while boosting your intake of omega-3s, -7s, and -9s. Most nutrition experts estimate that we eat about twenty times the omega-6s than omega-3s in our diet, which is not a healthy ratio. Omega-3s, which we need more of, are found in flaxseeds and hempseeds; omega-7s are primarily found in sea buckthorn berries, macadamia nuts, and to a lesser extent, fish. Omega-9s are primarily found in olives and olive oil, avocados, almonds, sesame oil, pecans, pistachios, cashews, hazelnuts, and macadamia nuts.

Myth #3: Safflower, canola, corn, and sunflower oils are good sources of omega-3s. **Fact**: These oils are highest in omega-6s, the ones you're most likely getting too much of. Even if you're not consciously aware of eating these oils, they are found in most baked goods and processed and prepared foods. That leads me to Myth #4.

Myth #4: Corn and canola oils are healthy. **Fact**: The crops these oils are derived from are heavily genetically modified, making any nutritional value they once held insufficient in comparison to the potential inflammation and health problems they may cause.

Myth #5: Fish is the only good source of omega-3 fatty acids. **Fact**: There are many excellent plant-based sources of omega-3 fatty acids. Omega-3 fatty acids are the equivalent of nutritional gold because they are nature's anti-inflammatory nutrients and are used in most chemical functions in the body. Although fatty fish are frequently considered the best source of this essential fatty acid, they are not the only source. Here are some excellent plant-based sources of omega-3s:

Blueberries: one cup of fresh blueberries contains 174mg of omega-3s.

Cashews: a one ounce serving of cashews contains 221mg of omega-3s.

Cauliflower: one cup of cooked cauliflower contains 208mg of omega-3s.

Chia seeds: one ounce of chia seeds contains 4915mg of omega-3s.

Flaxseeds: one ounce of flax seeds contains 6388mg of omega-3 fatty acids.

Hemp seeds: one ounce of hemp seeds provides 1100mg of omega-3s.

Honeydew melon: one cup of honeydew melon contains 58mg of omega-3s.

Mangoes: one mango contains 77mg of omega-3s.

Mustard oil: one tablespoon of mustard oil has 826mg of omega-3s; however, mustard oil should not be used in higher doses due to possible liver toxicity.

Pumpkin seeds: one quarter cup of pumpkin seeds contains 40mg of omega-3s.

Sesame Seeds: a one-ounce serving of sesame seeds contains 105mg of omega-3s.

Spinach: one cup of cooked spinach has 352mg of omega-3s.

Spirulina: one tablespoon of spirulina powder contains 58mg of omega-3s.

Tofu: one four-ounce serving of tofu contains 600mg of omega-3s.

Walnuts: one quarter cup of walnuts contains 2700mg of omega-3s.

Wild rice: one cup of cooked wild rice contains 156mg of omega-3s.

Winter squash: one cup of cooked squash contains 338mg of omega-3s.

Myth #6: All fish containing omega-3 fatty acids are suitable for consumption. **Fact**: Although there are many types of fish that contain high amounts of this omega-3 fatty acid–including mackerel, sardines, albacore tuna, salmon, lake trout, and herring–mackerel, tuna, and farm-raised salmon are often high in pollutants like mercury and are best avoided.

Myth #7: All packaged foods that contain omega-3 fatty acids are healthy. **Fact**: Most companies add omega-3 fatty acids to make otherwise unhealthy foods seem healthier. It has become a common practice for food manufacturers to add omega-3 fatty acids to their products. Consider that Breyers Smart! Yogurt contains a miniscule 32mg of the omega-3 known as DHA and one serving of Silk Soymilk Plus Omega-3 DHA contains only 32mg of DHA. For comparison's sake, one of the highest sources of omega-3 fatty acids, a six-ounce serving of salmon, contains more than one hundred times the amount of DHA found in these products.

THE TOP FOODS THAT FIGHT ALLERGIES

There are many naturally occurring plant compounds called phytonutrients that assist with allergies. The main ones include anthocyanins, curcumin, hesperetin, and quercetin. Don't worry about remembering their names or even pronouncing their names, as it is not necessary to do so to benefit from their antiallergy effects. I've listed the food sources of each below. Of course, if you have a food allergy or sensitivity to one of the sources indicated, avoid that food.

Eat Foods Rich in Anthocyanins

The phytonutrient group known as anthocyanins give foods their purplish-red color. They have natural anti-inflammatory properties. Anthocyanins are found in most dark red- and purple-colored foods, including beets, berries, cherries, and grapes.

Eat Curries to Benefit from Anti-inflammatory Curcumin

Turmeric (*Curcuma longa*) is a yellow-colored spice commonly found in Indian curries. It contains the active ingredient *curcumin*, which is a powerful antioxidant and anti-inflammatory substance. Research has shown that ingesting 1200mg of curcumin daily can have the same effect as anti-inflammatory drugs. You'd need to supplement to obtain that dose; however, you can also add fresh or dried turmeric to many foods, such as soups, curries, stews, salad dressings, and so forth. Be sure to avoid dairy-based curries, or you'll be undermining many of the anti-inflammatory benefits of turmeric, as dairy products are mucus forming.

Hesperetin/Hesperidin for Hay Fever

Hesperetin and hesperidin are almost identical except that the latter is bound to a sugar molecule. Research shows that these potent phytonutrients have antihistamine, antioxidant, anti-inflammatory, anticarcinogenic, and cholesterol-lowering actions, and they also protect blood vessels against damage—just a few of the many benefits of this healing nutrient. Hesperetin is found in the highest concentrations in green vegetables and citrus fruits like lemons and grapefruits, particularly in the white part, known as the pith. Of course, avoid citrus fruits if you suspect you are sensitive to them.

Take Quercetin to Quell Allergy Symptoms

When it comes to nutrients that prevent or treat allergies, it's hard to beat quercetin. This plant-based nutrient is best known for its ability to inhibit the release of histamine, the chemical responsible for the uncomfortable symptoms of seasonal allergies. Quercetin is a natural antihistamine that doesn't have the side effects of drowsiness, heartbeat irregularities, and other uncomfortable symptoms of the drug antihistamines that are commonly used. Additionally, quercetin is also a potent antioxidant that has anti-inflammatory effects, making it perfect for treating allergies and their effects on the body.

Research shows that eating a quercetin-rich diet reduces allergies and lowers LDL (harmful) cholesterol, blood pressure (when it is high), and risk of heart disease as well as the risk of prostate, colon, ovarian, breast, gastric, prostate, and cervical cancers. Some studies show that people who eat a lot of apples have improved lung function and a reduced risk of lung conditions, which is likely due, at least in part, to their high quercetin content.

Quercetin is classified as a flavonoid compound, which means this nutrient is responsible for the bright colors of many fruits and vegetables. Because it is an effective anti-inflammatory and antihistamine, it has been found to be an effective natural treatment for asthma due to allergies. It also helps alleviate nasal allergy symptoms.

Research in the medical journal *Acta BioMedica* found that a dietary supplement containing quercetin significantly improved both nasal and eye symptoms such as runny nose, sneezing, congestion, and sinus pressure.[25] Additional research in the journal *Cornea* found that quercetin helps alleviate dry eyes and regulate tear gland function.[26]

Brazilian animal research found that quercetin is also effective against asthma as a result of the nutrient's immune-modulating effects and ability to dilate the bronchial tubes.[27] Asthma is often triggered by pollens, dust, and other allergy-related substances. Quercetin also helps alleviate nasal allergy symptoms.

In one study, quercetin reduced histamine release in people with seasonal allergies by 96 percent. Take 400mg/day of quercetin with 100mg of bromelain and 500mg of vitamin C.[28]

There are many excellent sources of quercetin, including apples, blueberries, chives, cocoa powder, cranberries, lovage, onions, and tarragon. Additionally, some medicinal herbs are excellent sources of quercetin, including milk thistle, olive leaf, bilberry, elder, licorice, primrose, *Tribulus terrestris*, and motherwort. It's interesting to note that quercetin has been found to have mood-boosting properties as well, which could account for some of the mood-lifting herbs' benefits. Some of these quercetin-containing, mood-lifting herbs include St. John's wort, hops, valerian, passionflower, chamomile, and gingko. Here are some of the best food sources, along with the amount of quercetin in milligrams per one hundred grams of each food. All references are to cooked foods unless indicated otherwise:[29]

Ancho peppers: 27.6
Apples, raw with skin: 4.42
Apples, raw without skin: 1.5

Apricot, raw: 2.55

Black currants, raw: 5.69

Blueberries, frozen: 3.93

Broccoli, raw: 3.21

Buckwheat: 23.09

Buckwheat flour: 2.71

Capers, canned: 180.77

Chives, raw: 4.77

Cocoa powder, dry unsweetened: 20.13

Coriander, raw: 5.0

Cranberries, raw: 14.02

Cranberry juice, raw: 16.41

Dill, fresh: 55.15

Dock: 86.20

Hot green chili peppers, raw: 16.8

Hot wax yellow peppers, raw: 50.63

Jalapeno, raw: 5.07

Kale, raw: 7.71

Lemons, raw without peel: 2.29

Lingonberries, raw: 12.16

Lovage leaves: 170.0

Onions, boiled: 19.36

Red onion, raw: 19.93

Serrano peppers: 15.98

Spring onions, raw: 14.24

Tarragon, fresh: 10.0

Tea, black, brewed: 2.07

Tea, black, brewed decaf: 2.84

Tea, green, brewed: 2.69

Tea, green, brewed decaf: 2.77

Tomato puree: 4.12

Watercress, raw: 4.0

White sweet onion, raw: 5.19

Yellow snap beans, raw: 3.03

In addition to eating a high-quercetin diet, allergy sufferers frequently benefit from taking quercetin in supplement form to assist with allergy-induced sinus congestion, runny eyes or nose, or other allergy symptoms. Most people find relief from taking 400mg of quercetin twice daily.

To improve your absorption of quercetin, take it along with the enzyme bromelain, which is naturally present in raw pineapple, not cooked or canned pineapple. Alternatively, you can take it in capsule or tablet form. Many supplements formulated for allergies combine quercetin and bromelain to boost quercetin absorption. If you're in the midst of allergy season and already suffering from allergy symptoms, you may need up to 800mg of quercetin daily in divided doses. Read more about quercetin supplementation in chapter 5.

APPLES

Martin Luther once said, "Even if I knew that tomorrow the world would go to pieces, I would still plant my apple tree." New research gives more reasons than ever to plant apple trees and enjoy their delicious and nutritious fruit. Other than their sweet flavor, here are a few more reasons to sink your teeth into an apple today.

In studies, apples have been shown to significantly alter the amounts of the bacteria *Clostridiales* and *Bacteroides* in the large intestine, conferring gastrointestinal health benefits and reducing inflammation in the gut, which is linked to allergies.[30]

Thanks to their phytonutrient content, apples have been proven to lower the risk of asthma and other lung conditions in numerous studies.[31]

Apples contain multiple types of nutrients known as flavonoids, which have been shown to reduce allergy symptoms.

MORE GREAT ANTIALLERGY FOODS

Lemons

Although we already discussed that lemons contain the phyto-nutrient hesperetin, which has been shown in studies to alleviate allergic symptoms, they also contain a substance known as rutin, which has been shown in research to improve the symptoms of eye conditions, including those linked to allergies. Lemons also contain vitamin C, citric acid, flavonoids, B-complex vitamins, calcium, copper, iron, magnesium, phosphorus, potassium, and fiber.

Nettles

Most people are not aware that this common garden weed that rears its head in the springtime is a powerhouse of nutrition and an excellent addition to soups or stews. Nettles have been proven to reduce inflammation linked to allergies as well as seasonal allergy symptoms. If you're picking them yourself, be sure to find an experienced herbal guide and to wear thick gloves. Cooking destroys the stinging part of the plant, rendering it edible. For more information about nettles, see chapter 5.

PLENTY OF REASONS TO EAT ORGANIC FOOD

Organic food was the only option for thousands of years. Now with pesticides, herbicides, fungicides, and genetically modified foods, organic is still the best option and the best way to ensure allergy relief. Here are sixteen reasons to eat organic food:

1. Genetically modified foods were unleashed on the environment and the public by corporations without prior testing to determine their safety. In other words, eating genetically modified foods (which most people do in in large amounts)

is participating in a long-term, uncontrolled experiment. Choose organic to avoid participation in this experiment.

2. More and more research is coming in about the health threat of genetically modified food. The results range from intestinal damage, allergies, liver or pancreatic problems, testicular cellular changes, tumors, inflammation, and even death in the experimental animals. For more information, read the excellent books by Jeffrey M. Smith, *Seeds of Deception* and *Genetic Roulette*. Eating third-party-certified organic foods or those that are guaranteed to be grown from organic seed helps protect you from the health consequences of GMOs.

3. In study after study, research from independent organizations consistently shows that organic food is higher in nutrients than nonorganic foods. Research also shows that organic produce is higher in vitamin C, antioxidants, and the minerals calcium, iron, chromium, and magnesium.

4. They contain fewer neurotoxic organophosphates— neurotoxins are those toxins that are damaging to brain and nerve cells. A commonly used class of pesticides called organophosphates was originally developed as a toxic nerve agent during World War I. When there was no longer a need for them in warfare, industry adapted them to kill pests on foods. Many pesticides are still considered neurotoxins.

5. They're supportive of growing children's brains and bodies. Children's growing brains and bodies are far more susceptible to toxins than adults. Choosing organic helps feed their bodies without the exposure to pesticides and GMOs, both of which have a relatively short history of use—and, therefore, safety.

6. They are real food, not pesticide factories. Some genetically modified seeds and the foods grown from them are engineered to produce their own pesticides. I know it sounds more like science fiction than science fact, but it's

true. Sadly, once these seeds or foods are eaten, they may continue producing pesticides inside your body. Foods that are actually pesticide factories . . . no thanks.

7. Pesticides used in commercial agricultural practices frequently pollute our drinking water. Organic farming is the best solution to the problem. Buying organic helps reduce pollution in our drinking water.

8. Organic food is earth supportive—when Big Agra keeps its hands out of it. Organic food production has been around for thousands of years and is the sustainable choice for the future. Compare that to modern agricultural practices that destroy the environment through widespread use of herbicides, pesticides, fungicides, and fertilizers and have resulted in drastic environmental damage in many parts of the world.

9. Organic food choices grown on small-scale organic farms help ensure that independent family farmers can create a livelihood. Consider it the domestic version of fair trade.

10. Most organic food simply tastes better than the pesticide-grown counterparts.

11. Organic food is not exposed to gas-ripening like some nonorganic fruits and vegetables, such as bananas.

12. Organic farms are safer for farm workers. Research at the Harvard School of Public Health found a 70 percent increase in Parkinson's disease among people exposed to pesticides. Choosing organic foods means that more people will be able to work on farms without incurring the higher potential health risk of Parkinson's or other illnesses.

13. Organic food supports wildlife habitats. Even with commonly used amounts of pesticides, exposure to pesticides is harming wildlife.

14. Eating organic may reduce your cancer risk. The US Environmental Protection Agency (EPA) considers 60 percent of herbicides, 90 percent of fungicides, and 30 percent of

insecticides potentially cancer causing. It is reasonable to think that the rapidly increasing rates of cancer are at least partly linked to the use of these carcinogenic pesticides.

15. Choosing organic meat lessens your exposure to antibiotics, synthetic hormones, and drugs that are used in the rearing of nonorganic animals and, ultimately, end up in your body. These synthetic ingredients can throw off your gut's microbial balance.

16. Organic food supports greater biodiversity. Diversity is fundamental to life on this planet. Genetically modified and nonorganic food is focused on high-yield monoculture and is destroying biodiversity.

THE POWER OF WATER

Drink at least eight to ten cups of pure water daily to support the natural cleansing systems in your body. In my experience, I've found that staying well hydrated helps alleviate many allergy symptoms. I recommend filtering and alkalizing water to reduce harmful toxins found in water as well as to restore its naturally alkaline biochemistry. Prior to the Industrial Age and the many resulting pollutants as well as the process of adding chlorine and fluoride to water, water was naturally alkaline, which is the form of water best used by the body. The measurement of alkalinity is on a scale of zero to fourteen, with zero being extremely acidic and fourteen being extremely alkaline. Our cells need to maintain a largely alkaline state, and drinking alkaline water makes it much easier for them to do so. I've personally observed that switching to alkaline water can help reduce allergy symptoms. While there are many costly water alkalizing systems, I've found some excellent and affordable options ranging from a fifteen-dollar alkalizing stick to a two-hundred-dollar filtration and alkalizing system, and lots of options in between.

3

Addressing an Almost Unknown Cause of Allergies

F I ASKED YOU what one of the main causes of allergies is, you might tell me an overreactive immune system, an excess of pollens or dust, or a genetic predisposition toward allergies. And although these answers are all correct to a certain degree, it still begs the question: What causes some people's immune systems to overreact and to develop allergies to common, everyday substances? The answer might surprise you: the story of allergies begins in the gut.

KIMBERLY G. IMPROVES ALLERGIES AND ASTHMA WITH PROBIOTIC THERAPY

One of my readers sent me the following story about her experience with allergies and asthma: "I've had asthma and allergy problems all of my life. I have been able to manage it all naturally as research and information became more available. For me, I blame the allergies on antibiotics that had killed off the good bacteria. There has been some great research out there linking this. Because of it and after reading your book . . . I've begun to use probiotic therapy with great results! My allergies and asthma are subsiding!"

Like Kimberly, you can use probiotic therapy to improve one of the main causes of allergies and asthma: an unhealthy gut. Infections can cause an excessively permeable membrane in the gut, which is known as a leaky gut, and this in turn causes inflammation and toxins and microbes to enter the bloodstream, resulting in a hyperactive and imbalanced immune system. Et voilà: allergies. Using high doses of the allergy-fighting and gut-health-building strains of probiotics along with eating more fermented foods like sauerkraut, kimchi, yogurt (preferably vegan), and others can help eliminate infections, boost healthy microbes, and reduce inflammation in the gut, which helps alleviate allergies.

THE GUT CONNECTION

You may be surprised to learn that probiotics are among the best natural remedies for allergies. If you're hooked on antihistamines, decongestants, and desensitization shots, you might be inclined to think there is little value in such miniscule microbes, or you may believe that probiotics are purely beneficial for gut health. But more and more research shows that specific probiotic strains could be just the natural allergy remedy you've been waiting for. The reality is that there is a gut-allergy connection that few people are aware of. What happens in your gut determines the health of many other aspects of your body, including allergies.

The Gut-Allergy Connection

An unhealthy digestive tract is frequently the source of inflammation in the body, even inflammation that occurs somewhere seemingly unrelated, such as the sinuses or eyes. To help you understand the gut's link to inflammation and allergies, let's take a brief tour of the gastrointestinal (GI) tract.

Your Remarkable Gut

Although you may never give your gut a second thought unless you have indigestion or heartburn, it plays a critical role in your health. The food you eat contains proteins, carbohydrates, and fats, which the digestive tract breaks down into amino acids, sugars, and fatty acids, respectively. These compounds form the building blocks of all the cells, tissues, and organs in your body. Ideally the food you ingest also contains plentiful amounts of vitamins, minerals, and many other nutritional components such as enzymes (specialized proteins, phytonutrients), plant nutrients, and probiotics (beneficial bacteria and yeasts). We'll discuss probiotics in greater detail momentarily.

Although few people realize the importance of nutrients, the *Oxford Dictionary* definition of a vitamin is "any of a group of organic compounds which are essential for normal growth and nutrition and are required in small quantities in the diet because they cannot be synthesized by the body."[1] Minerals are inorganic substances found in food that are also essential to the functioning of the body and include calcium, magnesium, iron, and many others.

The digestive tract comprises many organs, including the mouth, salivary glands located in the mouth, stomach, small intestine, large intestine, liver, gall bladder, pancreas, as well as others, but these are the main ones we'll be discussing. The average person's GI tract is about twenty feet long and has the immense burden of processing approximately twenty-five tons of food over a person's lifetime. But it also serves many other important functions.

From the moment you put food into your mouth, digestion begins. The act of chewing begins the process of splitting the food apart to break it down into the building-block components

I mentioned earlier. The salivary glands start to secrete digestive juices full of enzymes that further break down the food, especially the starches and sugars found in the foods you eat.

The importance of chewing sufficiently cannot be overstated. The stomach and intestines cannot do the work of the teeth and the mouth. In other words, to sufficiently break down the food you eat into its essential compounds, you need to chew, chew, and chew some more.

After you swallow the food, it moves through a tube known as the esophagus until it reaches the stomach. In the stomach, the food sits for about twenty or thirty minutes, mixing with any enzymes secreted by the salivary glands as well as those found in the food. However, most of the food we eat has been heated, either during the cooking process or during manufacturing, well beyond the temperature at which enzymes can survive. At only 118 degrees Fahrenheit, which is not that hot at all, most enzymes in foods are destroyed and are no longer able to aid digestion.

After the enzymes in the food have mixed for up to half an hour, the food sustains an acid bath secreted by the stomach. The stomach acid works primarily to break down the food's protein compounds. The food then passes into the small intestine, where the nutrients that have been isolated during the digestive process are absorbed through villi in the intestinal wall and passed directly into the bloodstream. Villi are fingerlike protrusions that help absorb nutrients from food more efficiently. Once the nutrients and water from the food are absorbed through the walls of the intestines into the bloodstream, they travel to the places they are most needed. For example, calcium frequently travels through the intestinal walls into the blood and then to the nervous system, muscles, bones, or any other places calcium is used in the body to ensure proper functioning.

Even one nutrient deficiency can cause a wide range of problems in the body. But eating a healthy diet and popping nutritional supplements aren't the only ways to avoid nutrient deficiencies; it is also important to maintain healthy intestines. We'll discuss ways to do so momentarily.

Your liver, which sits below your lower ribs on the right side of your body, produces a green-colored liquid called bile and sends it to the gallbladder to be stored. The gallbladder then secretes bile as needed to assist with breaking down any fatty foods in your diet. The secretion of bile initiates contractions of the intestines to push any waste (left after the water and nutrients have been extracted from food) out of your large intestines.

We discussed some of the problems of the Standard American Diet in the last chapter, but it is important to note that this diet is deficient in many vitamins, minerals, other plant nutrients, enzymes, water, and fiber. Additionally, it is high in sugar, chemical additives, and preservatives, as well as inflammation-causing fats, to mention only a few of the many issues with such a diet. This type of diet tends to damage the villi protruding from the intestinal walls, making them less capable of absorbing nutrients from your food and supplements. Because of this, they frequently become inflamed and can even become blunt over time, which further impairs their ability to perform their nutrient extraction and absorption roles.

Inflammation of the intestinal walls, among other factors, can lead to an upset in the normal balance of beneficial to pathogenic microbes, a condition known as dysbiosis. This imbalance can cause harmful bacteria and yeasts to multiply, causing a wide range of negative symptoms, depending on the type of infections present. Dysbiosis can also increase the permeability of the intestinal walls, which may sound fine, but it is actually a serious concern. Harmful microbes can hijack the nutrient-absorption process and allow waste products and pathogenic microbes direct access to the bloodstream.

While medical scientists continue to search for the possible reasons some people have allergic responses to everyday pollens and other substances, further exploration of the gut-allergy connection will likely yield greater insights. In my experience and many years of research, I believe that dysbiosis is one of the primary causes of allergies and a wide range of other health concerns, including multiple sclerosis, celiac disease, and rheumatoid arthritis (check out my book *Arthritis-Proof Your Life*). Reinstating a low-allergen, anti-inflammatory diet while healing the gut and boosting the beneficial bacteria that reside there is a major step along the path to heal allergies.

WHY ALL THE FUSS ABOUT THE GUT?

Although Las Vegas may declare that "what happens in Vegas stays in Vegas," your gut takes the opposite approach. What happens in your gut does not stay there; instead, it spreads throughout your entire body to determine the health of almost every other bodily system including, at least in part, whether you suffer from allergies. Your gut plays a critical role in the health of your whole body. It is a factor in whether you'll experience allergies or even whether you will have a healthy immune system. Although many people are talking about the importance of gut health, few people realize that it is important to address the gut to deal with allergies.

Your body contains trillions of microorganisms—that's well beyond the number of cells in your entire body. Weighing about two pounds total, about 1 trillion of these microorganisms are stationed in your intestines. Your intestines contain approximately one thousand different species of bacteria. As Dr. Lynn Margulis, biologist and professor at the University of Massachusetts, Amherst, so aptly stated, "Life on earth is such a good story you cannot afford to miss the beginning . . . Beneath our superficial differences we are all of us walking communities of bacteria. The world shimmers, a pointillist landscape made up of tiny living beings."[2] Although we have been raised to believe that bacteria are the enemy—and some indeed may appear to be—most of the bacteria that reside in our bodies and our intestines in particular are of the friendly variety. Without them, we would not survive. Beneficial bacteria are essential to our health and, indeed, our life. If you've ever come across the medical term *microbiome*, it refers to the full collection of bacteria in your body, which is quite different from mine or anyone else's. Similar to fingerprints, no two people have exactly the same microbiome. There may be some similar types of bacteria, but they are not identical in variety or quantities of each.

Actually, as part of the Human Microbiome Project (HMP), scientists have been busy cataloging the many bacteria that live on or within the human body. Although this research is still under way, scientists have discovered that the bacteria on your left hand differ significantly from those on your right hand, which in turn differ extensively from those on the rest of your skin, which also differ from those in your intestines. And the bacteria on your right hand likely differ extensively from those found on mine. The scientists working on the HMP are primarily studying the bacteria in five sites on the human body, including the nasal passages, oral cavities, skin, GI tract, and urogenital tract. Although many other ecosystems exist in other areas of our body, they are simply focusing on these areas first.

As thanks for your hospitality in sharing your body with these beneficial bacteria, they contribute to many aspects of your health and life. Not only do they digest your food and manufacture nutrients you need to build healthy cells and tissues, but they also kill harmful disease-causing intruders. They even help regulate the production of compounds in your body that help boost your mood and help you feel free of anxiety and depression. And of course, they help lessen the likelihood you'll experience allergies.

If your next thought is similar to feedback I've had from readers and clients over the years, you may be thinking, *Well, I should be fine in the gut health department—after all, I eat yogurt.* Although yogurt may be a start in the right direction to help boost gut health and alleviate allergies, it is only a very small start, as you'll soon discover.

In addition to some of their vital roles I've already shared, it is essential to have high amounts of beneficial bacteria in your intestines to destroy harmful bacteria and fungi as well as to quell inflammation in your body and regulate the immune system. These are some of the areas in which probiotics truly shine.

Research even shows that probiotic bacteria are incredibly intelligent. They can not only recognize the disease-causing molecular patterns of harmful microbes; they can also manufacture and secrete proteins that destroy harmful infections. They even secrete anti-inflammatory compounds that affect the walls of the intestines, where inflammation usually begins in the body. Not only does that mean that they help regulate the immune system, which is usually overactive in people with allergies, but they can also reduce the likelihood that the immune system will overact in response to environmental triggers.

Additionally, because probiotic bacteria secrete substances that kill harmful infections, they are beneficial to allergy sufferers as well. Although we rarely think of allergies as a sign of infection, they frequently are. Candida yeasts, or fungi, are among the primary culprits when it comes to allergies and allergy symptoms. Even though there are various types of opportunistic infections that are known as *candida, Candida albicans* is the most common one. While it is commonly referred to as a yeast infection, it is actually more accurate to refer to it as a fungal infection.

Here are some of the signs of a harmful intestinal overgrowth of either the bacterial or yeast variety:[3]

- allergies and food sensitivities
- anxiety
- autoimmune disorders (rheumatoid arthritis, lupus, Hashimoto's thyroiditis, fibromyalgia, etc.)

- back pain
- bad breath, gum disease, or dental problems
- belching
- bloating
- chronic fatigue
- constipation
- cramping or abdominal pain
- diarrhea
- difficulty losing weight
- diverticulitis/diverticulosis
- eczema or psoriasis
- flatulence
- heartburn or acid reflux
- high cholesterol levels
- indigestion
- irritable bowel syndrome (IBS)
- joint inflammation and stiffness
- nausea
- poor digestion
- poor sleep
- sinus infections
- sugar cravings
- yeast infections or vaginitis

The above list is by no means exhaustive. It is possible to have only a few of the above symptoms and still have an intestinal infection or bacterial or yeast overgrowth.

HOW TO HEAL A LEAKY GUT

Of the approximately thousand varieties of bacteria present in your gut, there are two types known as *Bifidobacteria* and *Bacteroides*. Research shows that these species of probiotics tend to be markedly reduced as we age.[4] A reduction in these and other beneficial bacteria can set the stage for improper immune sensing by the lymphoid tissue in the gut, also known as gut-associated lymphoid tissue (GALT), which leads to increased inflammation and intestinal permeability, frequently referred to as "leaky gut syndrome."

Not only can a reduction in beneficial bacteria lead to leaky gut syndrome, but excessive amounts of harmful bacteria can also cause the condition in which the intestinal walls become increasingly permeable. Instead of simply allowing water and nutrients to pass through the intestinal walls, small holes in the intestinal walls allow intestinal contents—including harmful bacteria, viruses, toxins, food particles, or intestinal waste—to travel across the wall, where they directly enter the bloodstream and make us vulnerable to inflammation, immune conditions, and many other health problems, including allergies. The immune system, sensing that these foreign materials should not be present in the blood, goes on high alert and begins to overwork as it attacks and attempts to eliminate them. The gut not only becomes inflamed, but low-grade inflammation also develops in weakened areas of the body and can spread over time.

Additionally, the gut's ability to absorb nutrients like vitamin B12, magnesium, iron, zinc, and others becomes impaired, leaving you feeling tired and irritable at first but prone to developing serious health issues over time, including an impaired immune system, which can overreact to environmental substances that it would not otherwise react to.

There are other causes of a leaky gut besides low counts of beneficial bacteria or high amounts of harmful bacteria or yeasts. Some other causes include chronically high levels of stress; toxins we're exposed to in our air, water, or food; inflammatory foods like sugar, dairy products, or high amounts of animal protein in our diet; pharmaceutical drugs; and other infections like viruses, among others. Additionally, if you eat a low-fiber diet or don't drink sufficient water daily, fecal matter, along with other substances it contains, can irritate the intestinal lining or cause the intestines to become misshapen from long-term constipation.

A leaky gut not only affects the gut but can impact the whole body as well. Symptoms of a leaky gut include bloating, cramping, fatigue, food sensitivities, flushing, achy joints, headaches, rashes, sinus congestion, and—you guessed it—allergies.

To fully address allergies for long-term health and recovery, it is imperative to address gut health to help the body to heal from a leaky gut.

A multifaceted approach to healing the gut tends to work best:

- Eliminate foods that cause inflammation, have insufficient fiber, or contain harmful food additives and refined sugar.
- Add healing, anti-inflammatory foods to the diet to help repair the gut and reduce inflammation throughout the body. Some of these foods include almond, cashew, coconut, or other plant-based yogurt with live cultures; sauerkraut with live cultures; other fermented vegetables or beverages; raw sprouts such as bean sprouts; sprouted seeds such as chia, flax, or hempseeds; and coconut foods like coconut oil, unsweetened coconut, coconut milk, and so forth.
- Add nutrients, herbs, and supplements that soothe the lining of the GI tract and repair the perforations involved in a leaky gut.[5] Some of these supplements include aloe vera juice, enzymes, L-glutamine, licorice root, and quercetin. Aloe vera juice is an excellent choice to soothe and heal the intestinal lining. Enzymes help ensure foods are fully digested to prevent whole food molecules from crossing through the gut wall into the

blood stream. L-glutamine is a natural amino acid found in protein that helps heal the gut wall while coating cells to help them repel irritants. Licorice root helps counter the harmful effects of stress and heals the gut walls. Quercetin restores the gut barrier by sealing the gut walls and, at the same time, reducing the body's release of histamine, which is linked to allergy symptoms.

• Supplement with gut-healing probiotics that boost beneficial bacteria, kill harmful bacteria and yeasts, and reduce inflammation, which I'll discuss in greater detail momentarily.

THE BEST PROBIOTICS FOR ALLERGIES

In addition to taking probiotics to prevent or treat dysbiosis, to heal a leaky gut, and to reduce inflammation in the gut or elsewhere in the body, some probiotic strains have been found to have specific antiallergic properties.

The ideal time to take probiotics to prevent allergies altogether is during gestation, infancy, or early childhood, but obviously this is not possible for most people, particularly as little was known about the health-giving properties of probiotics during our childhood years. But for those of you who may be looking out for the health of little ones, ensuring that they get probiotics early in life can help prevent allergies later on. There are specific formulations that are suitable for the mother to take during pregnancy or that can be included in children's food in childhood years. Be sure the product you choose is suitable. Little is known about how many of the probiotic strains intended for adults may affect childhood health.

According to research in the *Journal of Allergy and Clinical Immunology*, scientists found that probiotic consumption by the mother during pregnancy and in the infant's milk during infancy reduced the risk of allergy-induced eczema. Such early probiotic consumption also reduced the likelihood of allergy-related nasal and eye inflammation.[6] Known as allergic rhino-conjunctivitis (ARC), this common allergic condition involves inflammation of the nose, sinuses, and eyes. If you're an allergy sufferer, you're probably no stranger to the itchy nose, sneezing, watery mucus, nasal congestion or blockage, and itching or burning eyes involved in ARC.

Of course, for most allergy sufferers, it is no longer possible to consider fetal or infant nutrition. So what works after you're fully developed and have full-blown allergies? Probiotics can still help. Scientists at the Osaka University School of Medicine in Japan found that certain probiotics are beneficial in treating allergic symptoms. These probiotics also effectively reduced sinusitis and nasal congestion linked to allergies.[7] According to their study published in the *International Archives of Allergy and Immunology*, the specific strains that demonstrated effectiveness against allergy symptoms include *Lactobacilli casei*, *Lactobacillus paracasei*, *L. acidophilus*, and *Bifidobacterium longum*.

Although most people think probiotics are simply good bacteria, that is only part of the truth. Whereas the bulk of probiotics are bacteria, they aren't the only microbes that can help allergy sufferers. Other research in the medical journal *Advanced Therapeutics* found that the probiotic yeast known as *Saccharomyces cerevisiae* effectively reduces inflammation in the mucous membranes as well as acts as a nasal decongestant.[8] *S. cerevisiae* was also found to reduce congestion and runny noses. This beneficial yeast is not linked to yeast infections, which are caused by completely different yeast strains.

You may be tempted to think, *Well, I'm already taking a probiotic supplement.* But bear in mind that not all probiotics offer relief. Some strains do nothing at all to reduce allergies but may be helpful for other health conditions. It is important to choose one or more of the above science-backed strains, as they have been found effective against allergies specifically rather than just taking a shotgun approach.

Additionally, for probiotics to work to alleviate allergies, it is imperative to take them daily to help the beneficial microbes build up in the body to reduce inflammation and allergy symptoms. Although probiotics can start working on allergy symptoms immediately, they also tend to build up in the body over time. Don't discount them if you don't get immediate improvement in symptoms. They work by going to the root cause of the condition rather than just slapping a Band-Aid on symptoms, so it may take time to notice improvements.

Supplement your diet with a high-quality probiotic taken on an empty stomach, preferably one containing a wide variety of bacterial strains. Don't worry about remembering their lengthy names. Usually the word *Lactobacillus* will be shortened to *L.*, and *Bifidobacterium* will be shortened to *B.* on product labels.

Usually bacteria are measured in colony-forming units—CFU for short—and most types will have between 1 and 20 billion CFU. Or the package may just indicate, say, 4 billion per capsule. However, don't be fooled into thinking that choosing a quality probiotic is just a numbers game. Unfortunately, there isn't a good way to discern between good- and poor-quality probiotic supplements without trying them or reviewing consumer studies. To learn more about which probiotic products measure up and which ones don't, check out my book *The Probiotic Promise*.

By taking a broad-spectrum probiotic supplement that includes *Lactobacilli casei*, *Lactobacillus paracasei*, *L. acidophilus*, *Bifidobacterium longum*, and *Saccharomyces cerevisiae*, you'll increase your likelihood of reducing allergy symptoms. Probiotic supplements work over time. Do not expect to see immediate results like you would with certain other supplements. Take probiotic supplements on an empty stomach and away from antibiotics or oregano oil supplements. For most people, the ideal time is either before bed or first thing in the morning. If you take it in the morning, try to leave at least twenty to thirty minutes before eating.

The dosage varies depending on the product selected. Follow package directions. If your allergy symptoms persist and you're following the dietary plan outlined earlier, double the recommended dosage. You may initially experience some bloating, flatulence, and increased bowel movements as your body adjusts to the higher dosage. This is the result of the beneficial bacteria and yeasts killing harmful microbes in your intestines. These symptoms usually subside in several days. Pregnant or nursing women should only use probiotic supplements intended for pregnancy at the recommended dose.

FERMENTED FOODS THAT HELP ALLEVIATE ALLERGIES

One of the best ways to obtain more beneficial probiotics that help alleviate allergies is to enjoy more fermented foods like non-dairy yogurt, sauerkraut, kimchi, kefir, and cultured vegetables. Not only do these foods boost the number and diversity of probiotics in our bodies; they also help heal a leaky gut, reduce inflammation, and alleviate the incidence and severity of allergies when eaten regularly over time. And who knows? You may find some new favorite foods in the process of experimenting with more fermented foods. Both my husband and I did. As we explored fermented vegetables, different types of vegan yogurts, fermented juices and teas, as well as kimchi, we've found many foods that we love so much, we want to include them in our diet regularly.

Sauerkraut

Who hasn't enjoyed sauerkraut on a hot dog or sausage? That's how most of us have tried sauerkraut for the first time. But there's more reason than ever to enjoy this tart, fermented food:

new and exciting research demonstrates the many healing properties of eating naturally fermented sauerkraut regularly, including its antibacterial and antifungal properties, including against Candida, as well as its ability to reduce allergy symptoms.

The Division of Sports Medicine at the University of Hawai'i at Mānoa in Honolulu reviewed probiotic-rich foods including sauerkraut in their research on athletic performance. Published in *Current Sports Medicine Reports*, the scientists found that numerous health benefits were attributable to probiotic-rich foods on athletic performance, including reducing allergic conditions and enhancing recovery from fatigue as well as improving immune function.[9] Regardless of whether you're a professional athlete or a weekend warrior, you may want to take note of the power of fermented foods like sauerkraut to reduce allergy symptoms while enhancing your athletic performance.

And like the German versions of this delicious and nutritious food, the Asian versions that typically use Chinese cabbage also offer many health benefits. In a study published in the journal *Evidence-Based Complementary and Alternative Medicine*, scientists at the National Taipei University of Education found that Taiwanese fermented cabbage regulated the immune system of mice and even demonstrated the ability to reduce or prevent allergic reactions. They concluded that Taiwanese fermented cabbage offers promise for the treatment of allergic diseases.[10] I'm sure that German sauerkraut offers similar results.

Unfortunately, most commercially sold sauerkraut doesn't contain any beneficial probiotics. Many commercial sauerkraut manufacturers have taken shortcuts in the making of sauerkraut to increase their profits. Instead of waiting for natural fermentation to occur, many instead employ an artificial pickling-type process that uses white vinegar, which doesn't contain any probiotics. And those companies that do stay true to natural processes still frequently pasteurize their sauerkraut so it can remain on grocery store shelves for longer periods. This pasteurization or heating process during bottling kills any live cultures that are needed for the health benefits of sauerkraut. Choose only sauerkraut with live cultures found in the refrigerator section of your health food or grocery store. Better yet, it is easy to make your own at home. For more information on how to make sauerkraut, check out my book *The Probiotic Promise*.

Kimchi

You've probably never given kimchi consideration when you think of ways to improve allergies, but you might want to enjoy kimchi regularly, given the exciting research into kimchi's healing properties.

A growing body of research has shown that kimchi can play an important role in alleviating allergy symptoms. A study published in the *Journal of Clinical Immunology* found that certain lactobacilli bacteria found in kimchi could reduce the overreaction of the airways in the lungs when animal lungs were exposed to allergens. *Lactobacillus plantarum* and *Lactobacillus curvatus* bacteria both demonstrated the greatest reduction of allergen-induced lung reactions.[11]

Although the incidence of allergies linked to kimchi consumption has not been studied to the best of my knowledge, I think it would prove to be beneficial in this area as well.

There are many varieties of kimchi, which vary greatly from region to region and even household to household, depending on the person or company making this fermented food.

Kefir

Few people have even heard about kefir, which is similar to a thinner, drinkable form of yogurt. Like yogurt, it is typically a fermented milk product, although I am more inclined to recommend the nondairy and juice varieties of this beverage for allergy sufferers. Kefir has a tart, tangy, and somewhat sour taste and a slight effervescence. The word *kefir* comes from the Turkish word *keif*, which I understand means "good feeling," probably due to the health benefits it confers. Kefir is believed to have three times the overall number of probiotics than yogurt and about ten to twenty different bacteria and yeast strains, where yogurt might have only two or three.

A study published in the *Brazilian Journal of Microbiology* found that kefir and its constituents have antimicrobial and immune system–regulating activity.[12] As if that wasn't enough, additional research shows that kefir consumption may offer hope for allergy and asthma sufferers as well.[13]

Miso

Miso is a fermented bean paste that is typically made from soybeans, although there are rice and chickpea misos as well. Most people are only familiar with its use in miso soup, but it is used as a flavoring in salad dressings as well as the making of many artisanal vegan cheeses. The *Journal of Allergy and Clinical Immunology* found that the more miso the participants ingested, the lower their symptoms of allergic rhinitis (nasal congestion due to allergies).[14]

Miso is rich in minerals, vitamins, protein, good carbs, enzymes, and probiotics. Heating miso, like any other food rich in enzymes or probiotics, destroys both, so it is best to enjoy miso in an unheated form rather than the traditional miso soup.

Yogurt

Before you grab that decongestant to subdue your sinus congestion or that antihistamine to stop the sneezing linked to spring allergies, you might want to give your gut some attention by eating more vegan yogurt. Although dairy-based yogurt may have many health-building properties, like other dairy products, it is highly mucus forming and should be avoided if you have allergies. Fortunately, there are many excellent vegan yogurt options like coconut yogurt, almond yogurt, and cashew yogurt. And as you learned earlier, more and more research shows that probiotics like those found in fermented foods like yogurt can help alleviate allergy symptoms and may even prevent allergic conditions altogether if they are started early in life. Because it can help heal the gut, leaky gut included, enjoying yogurt daily can help address the root causes of allergies. Some of the probiotics in yogurt also help reduce inflammation, which is just one more way yogurt consumption can help with allergies.

EIGHT TIPS TO BUY BETTER YOGURT

Despite all the hype, not all yogurt is good for you. Here are eight tips to help you select the best and healthiest yogurt for you:

1. Look for live cultures. The live cultures in yogurt provide the many beneficial gut health and overall health benefits we attribute to yogurt. So be sure to look for a yogurt that says "live cultures" on the package. It could be in the ingredients list or somewhere else on the package, but it needs to be there.

2. Check the sugar content. Some yogurt contains a whopping twenty-six to twenty-nine grams of sugar for an individual serving of yogurt. That's more than many soft drinks or doughnuts. Most of the sugars naturally present in milk or milk alternatives should be eliminated during the culturing process, as the sugars act as food for the probiotic cultures. If the yogurt contains much sugar, that means either (a) the manufacturer added sugar to the yogurt after the culturing process or (b) the culturing process didn't take place and the manufacturer added flavors and thickening agents to the milk instead.

3. Check the serving size. Some brands of yogurt list the amount of nutrients and sugars for a four-ounce serving, whereas others indicate a six- or eight-ounce serving size. That way you can compare the amount of sugar and nutrients based on similar servings.

4. Avoid any yogurt that says it has been "heat treated" after the culturing process or during the packaging process. The beneficial

probiotics that proliferate during the yogurt-making process are heat sensitive. If they are heated during packaging or at another stage of the manufacturing process, it is unlikely you will reap any of the health benefits of eating the yogurt. This type of product is better left at the store.

5. Avoid yogurt with fillers. Making yogurt takes two ingredients: a type of milk (or milk alternative) and live cultures. The cultures do the rest of the work to transform the milk into yogurt. If the yogurt you purchase contains more ingredients than just milk and live cultures, it probably contains harmful ingredients like sugar, colors, fillers, or other less-than-healthy substances and is best avoided.

6. Go Greek. When it comes to yogurt varieties, Greek or plain yogurt are preferable. That's because most of these varieties contain fewer ingredients like colors, fillers, or sweeteners.

7. Dairy-free yogurt is the best choice for allergy and asthma sufferers. In my research, I found that dairy-free yogurt varieties often contained a greater diversity of probiotic strains than dairy yogurt. That doesn't mean all dairy-free yogurt is better than cow's-milk yogurt, but it does mean you can still reap the health benefits of yogurt even while avoiding the dairy varieties.

8. If you're choosing cow's-milk yogurt, choose organic as much as possible. Cow's milk frequently contains antibiotics or other medication residues as well as the genetically modified hormone known as rBST. BST is a hormone known as bovine somatotropin; rBST is a genetically modified version of the hormone developed by Monsanto by using genetically engineered *E. coli* bacteria and is probably not something you want in your body.

Of course, there are no hard and fast rules, as there are many manufacturing and processing variables that determine the quality of the yogurt you choose, but the above guidelines will help you pick the best one for your buck.

As you learned earlier, GI infections can play a causative role in allergies. A study published in the *Journal of the American College of Nutrition* assessed the effects of yogurt consumption of a product containing live *L. casei* cultures on common GI infections in shift workers. The researchers found that the yogurt consumption could reduce the risk of GI infections.[15] In other research, yogurt was found to be effective against the nasty *H. pylori* bacteria, which has been linked to various gastrointestinal concerns. According to research published in the *World Journal of Gastroenterology*, yogurt consumption helps fight *H. pylori* infections.[16]

Consuming yogurt also increases the quantity of nutrients absorbed from other foods eaten at the same meal. A study in the *International Journal of Food Sciences and Nutrition* found that yogurt consumption increased the absorbability of other nutrients found in soy milk when the two foods were eaten at the same morning meal.[17] Of course, fermented soy yogurt likely has the same effect. If you eat soy products, be sure to choose only ones that are certified to be free of GMOs.

4

Enzymes—Miracle Warriors Against Allergies

MOST OF US ARE aware that we are more than a collection of bones, joints, muscles, cells, and other physical structures. Although these bodily parts are obviously important, as are the many biochemical processes that occur within our bodies, we are not simply the sum of these parts and processes; indeed, there is a spark that initiates and organizes processes within our body to keep us alive, functioning, and healthy. From a biochemical viewpoint, that spark comes in the form of enzymes, specialized forms of proteins that ensure every cellular and biochemical process can occur in the body. Enzymes act as catalysts to initiate, activate, or expedite virtually every process in the body. Unlike other types of protein molecules, enzymes are biologically active; in other words, they contain life force energy that act as sparks to awaken and incite the various processes in the body. We could not live without enzymes.

Extensive research by one of the earliest enzymologists, Dr. Edward Howell, revealed that enzyme shortages are commonly seen in people suffering from chronic diseases, including allergies, arthritis, premature aging, cancer, heart disease, skin conditions, and obesity.

Enzymes are used in vast quantities in our bodies to quell inflammation, promote healing, and regenerate tissues, which are all essential processes involved in allergies. So it should come as no surprise that poor food choices, an unhealthy lifestyle, or illness and injury may deplete our body's ability to manufacture sufficient enzymes to ensure these processes occur smoothly and to aid healing.

There are three main types of enzymes: metabolic, digestive, and food enzymes.

1. **Metabolic enzymes**—Metabolic enzymes are made by the body to properly run all its biochemical processes, from moving and talking to breathing and thinking. Each one of these enzymes has a unique function for which it is created. If any particular metabolic enzyme is missing or deficient in the body, it can lead to any number of serious diseases. Potentially thousands of life-supporting metabolic processes may suffer if there is a deficiency of enzymes in the body.

2. **Digestive enzymes**—Digestive enzymes assist with breaking down foods into their nutrient components for proper absorption. They are also called pancreatic enzymes because they are primarily secreted by the pancreas, an organ found just under the lower left side of your rib cage. The pancreas regulates blood sugar levels through the production and secretion of a hormone called insulin. It also manufactures and secretes more than twenty enzymes that are essential to digestion, including amylase, lipase, and protease enzymes. These enzymes digest carbohydrates, fats, and proteins, respectively.

3. **Food enzymes**—These enzymes, sometimes called plant enzymes, are found in raw plants such as fruits, vegetables, nuts, seeds, and herbs. By eating a diet rich in plant enzymes, you will dramatically reduce the number of digestive enzymes your body needs to manufacture, thereby freeing up energy and making more enzymes available to the body for healing. Eating plentiful amounts of foods rich in enzymes can not only give your energy a boost and help reduce the energy and enzymes needed for digestion but also boost the healing functions in the body.

The Standard American Diet (SAD) contains almost no enzymes other than perhaps those found in that piece of iceberg lettuce, slice of tomato, and sprinkling of onions found on a hamburger—certainly not enough to digest that meal and definitely none left over for healing.

Although there is little known at this time as to how we can support the production of adequate amounts of metabolic enzymes, we can improve digestion to reduce the burden on digestive enzymes. Additionally, there are two primary ways we can boost the necessary enzymes in the body:

1. Eat a diet rich in enzymes.
2. Supplement with additional enzymes that specifically work on inflammation reduction, balancing the immune system, and other relevant processes linked to allergies.

Before we discuss how to boost enzymes in the body, let's look at the effects of inadequate enzymes in the diet. Dr. Francis Pottenger Jr., MD, published the results of a study he conducted many years ago. He wanted to explore the damage of eating a diet devoid of enzymes to determine the effects of doing so on our body's own enzyme stores. He studied six hundred cats, feeding them a diet of food completely devoid of enzymes. The first generation of cats started suffering from "heart problems; nearsightedness; farsightedness; under activity of the thyroid or inflammation of the thyroid gland; infection of the kidney, of the liver, of the testes, of the ovaries; arthritis, inflammation of the joints; inflammation of the nervous system with paralysis and meningitis."[1]

The next generation of cats had symptoms that were worse than their parents'. Dr. Pottenger found that they were "much more irritable, dangerous to handle, sex interest is slack or perverted, role reversal, allergies, and skin lesions." Whereas about 25 percent of the cats born to the first generation died, Dr. Pottenger noted that 70 percent of the cats born to the second generation died. The deliveries were more difficult, and more of the pregnant cats died in labor.

The third generation of kittens suffered from similar health conditions. None lived past six months, and as a result, they were unable to produce offspring. There was no fourth generation of cats.

For comparison's sake, Dr. Pottenger fed another group of cats an enzyme-rich diet of raw meat, raw milk, and cod liver oil because cats are carnivorous animals. He observed healthy cats from one generation to the next.

Dr. Pottenger's study demonstrates that a shortage of enzymes in the cats' diets played a significant role in their health—or lack of it.

BOOSTING ENZYMES

In addition to eating a healthy diet like the one outlined in chapter 2, the best ways to boost the availability of enzymes for healing is to reduce the amount required for digestion, incorporate enzyme-rich foods into your diet, and either add supplementary enzymes either to meals or take them on an empty stomach, depending on the purpose of taking them. I'll discuss enzyme supplementation momentarily.

REDUCING THE DIGESTIVE BURDEN

Digestion requires plentiful amounts of the body's enzymes, particularly when we eat a diet high in animal protein, harmful fats, sugars, and other difficult-to-digest foods. We eat complex meals of meat, potatoes, gravy, and vegetables (maybe!), and then we top it all off with a wheat-, dairy-, and sugar-rich dessert, giving little consideration to the burden this type of meal or something similar puts on our digestive enzymes. This type of eating pattern in the SAD is enzyme intensive; in other words, it requires a vast number of enzymes produced by the body for adequate digestion. And our enzyme systems can easily become overwhelmed when we eat these heavy, complex meals regularly: think indigestion, bloating, and heaviness, and you'll have a good idea how much your digestive system may be struggling with these food choices. Check out "Eight Easy Ways to Improve Your Digestion" for ways to improve your digestion.

EIGHT EASY WAYS TO IMPROVE YOUR DIGESTION

1. Chew, chew, chew your food. Then chew it some more. As you may recall, enzymes in foods are released by chewing them well. Plus, chewing well allows food to mingle longer with your salivary juices, helping break them down further and ensuring more digestion occurs in the upper chamber of the stomach.

2. Don't drink with meals. Or if you have supplements to take with meals, drink a small amount of water. Not only does drinking

with meals dilute the enzymes in your food and your body's digestive juices; it also prematurely raises the pH of your stomach—the signal that tells your stomach to dump stomach contents into the duodenum. That means undigested foods will prematurely find their way to your intestines, where they may cause inflammation or leak through the intestinal walls—a precursor to many illnesses.

3. Simplify your meals. Heavy, complex meals like a steak, baked potato, gravy, cake, and ice cream are harder to digest than simpler, lighter ones. Digestion requires a tremendous amount of energy and enzymes. Take the burden off your body by simplifying your diet.

4. Try not to eat when you are stressed out. If you are always stressed, learn some stress-management techniques. You're the only person who can manage the stress in your life. Emotional distress diverts a substantial amount of energy needed for digestion.

5. Eat prior to 7:00 or 7:30 p.m. That gives your body time to digest foods thoroughly before going to bed. If you work night shifts, avoid eating for at least three hours before bed. That means no late-night snacks. It also means you can take a probiotic supplement on an empty stomach before bed (refer back to item number two in this list).

6. Add a full-spectrum digestive enzyme to your meals. I'll discuss more about supplementing with enzymes later in this chapter.

7. Eat more fermented foods like sauerkraut, yogurt (preferably dairy-free options), kimchi, kombucha (a fermented tea beverage), and others. Be sure they contain live cultures. You'll find these foods in the refrigerator section of your health food or grocery store. For more information about fermented foods, check out my book *The Probiotic Promise* as well as my blog on CulturedCook.com.

8. Replenish enzymes in your diet. That means eating more foods in their natural, uncooked state, such as raw fruits, vegetables, nuts, and seeds.

REPLENISHING OUR ENZYME-DEPLETED DIET

As you learned in chapter 2, our so-called modern diet is replete with many weaknesses: it is high in trans fats, saturated fats, sugar, chemical food additives, sodium, and less-than-desirables. And it contains insufficient amounts of vitamins, minerals, essential fatty acids, phytonutrients, and enzymes.

Fruits, vegetables, nuts, and seeds are replete with their own enzymes to digest them if eaten in a raw, natural state. But most enzymes are destroyed at 118 degrees Fahrenheit, which is not very hot at all. When the enzymes are destroyed, the food will no longer contain all the enzymes needed to digest it and will instead deplete your body's own digestive enzymes. Most of our foods are cooked well beyond that temperature, destroying all the enzymes they once contained.

It's not necessary to eat all your foods in a raw state, but you can see the problem when you eat almost no raw fruits, vegetables, nuts, or seeds: your body has to pick up the slack, depleting your digestive enzymes in the process. Not only does this result in reduced digestive function and more symptoms of indigestion; many digestive enzymes also double as metabolic enzymes that can reduce inflammation and help heal the joints when they are not needed to digest food.

Most of us fry, sauté, bake, broil, barbecue, microwave, or steam our foods, ensuring that any enzymes that may be present in the food are destroyed in the cooking process. Simply making an effort to obtain more raw foods in your diet can make a difference to improve your health. You may be having visions of rabbit food just now, but it's not necessary to eat like a rabbit to enjoy more raw foods and the health benefits they offer. I absolutely love delicious gourmet foods, and I wouldn't eat like a rabbit, but I eat a high amount of raw foods regularly.

You may be thinking that you find it hard to digest raw fruits and vegetables. If you are one of the people who find these foods difficult to digest, you are simply not chewing your food adequately. These foods contain all the enzymes they need to be digested comfortably and completely, but the enzymes need to be broken down to be accessible. The way to break them down is to chew them well.

Here are some easy ways to enjoy more raw foods in your diet:

- Eat more fruit in its natural state. Instead of pastries or processed sweets, indulge your sweet tooth with some delicious fruit. Enjoy some pineapple, apples, pomegranates, cherries, blueberries, and other delicious fruits. Once you make it a habit, you'll find you won't miss other sweets anyway.
- Snack on vegetable crudité with hummus or a dairy-free veggie dip.
- Eat at least one leafy green salad every day. There are dozens of possible ingredients you can use to keep it interesting and delicious. To help you get started, check out the text box "Create a Gourmet, Health-Building Salad in Minutes" on page 83.
- Enjoy fermented foods like dairy-free yogurt, sauerkraut, kimchi, kombucha (fermented tea), and others. Make sure the ones you choose say *live cultures* so they contain beneficial bacteria and health-supporting yeasts that boost enzymes and digestion.
- Snack on raw, unsalted nuts that have been soaked in water for a few hours. Soaking them ahead of time deactivates enzyme inhibitors found in the nuts. I set out a couple of bowls of nuts in water at night before heading to bed so they'll be ready to snack on the next day.

CREATE A GOURMET, HEALTH-BUILDING SALAD IN MINUTES

If you avoid salads at any cost, thinking they consist only of iceberg lettuce and a couple of slices of starchy tomato topped with some chemical- and sugar-laden bottled dressing, you will be happy to learn that with minimal effort you can create salads that inspire health *and* your taste buds.

These excellent salads can be gourmet meals in themselves. The idea is to be creative. This list is just to help you get started.

SALAD BASES

beets (grated)

boston lettuce

brown rice (cooked)

endive

grated cabbage

leaf lettuce

mixed greens

parsley

quinoa (cooked)

radicchio

romaine lettuce

seaweed, such as arame, nori, or wakami

sprouts, such as alfalfa, mung bean, or red clover

watercress

wild rice

MIX-INS

alfalfa sprouts

apples (sliced or grated)

avocado

beets (grated)

bell peppers (red, green, or yellow)

blackberries

blueberries

broccoli (finely chopped)

broccoli sprouts

carrots (julienned, roasted, or grated)

celery

celery root

chickpeas

cucumber slices

edible flowers, such as
    nasturtiums, violas,
    or pansies

fenugreek sprouts

grapefruit slices

great northern beans

kidney beans

lima beans

mung bean sprouts

mushrooms (raw or cooked)

olives

onion (minced)

onion sprouts

orange slices

pea shoots

peas (fresh)

pinto beans

pomegranate seeds

radishes

raspberries

red clover sprouts

scallions

strawberries

sweet potato (grated or roasted)

tomatoes

zucchini (grated or roasted)

TOPPINGS

almond slices

carrots (grated)

fresh basil (chopped)

fresh cilantro
    (chopped)

fresh mint (chopped)

fresh parsley (chopped)

hazelnuts (chopped)

herbs (such as thyme, oregano,
    minced garlic)

pine nuts

pumpkin seeds

sesame seeds

sunflower seeds

DRESSINGS

balsamic vinegar

oil and lemon juice

olive oil

your favorite homemade dressing

SUPPLEMENTING WITH ENZYMES

There's good reason to consider adding enzyme supplements to your allergy-proof program: they work. You can supplement your diet with a high-quality, full-spectrum digestive enzyme formula that includes amylase, lipase, and protease, among other enzymes, which break down starches and sugars, fats, and protein, respectively, the major building blocks of foods. The approach of taking enzymes with meals is beneficial for your digestion and overall energy levels. But there is an even better way of taking enzymes to alleviate allergy symptoms and aid healing: *systemic enzyme therapy.*

Systemic enzyme therapy—the use of enzyme supplements taken on an empty stomach is the natural medicine of the future when it comes to allergies and many other health conditions. The same enzymes that would normally act on the foods you eat instead go to work on reducing swelling such as that in the sinuses and nasal passageways during allergy season, eliminating the by-products of inflammation, dissolving mucus, and boosting the healing of the immune system.

Supplementing your diet with a high-quality, full-spectrum digestive enzyme formula that includes the amylase, lipase, protease, and other enzymes is beneficial for digestion and gut health. Take one to three enzyme capsules or tablets with every meal to help your body break down the carbohydrates, fats, and proteins in your food into natural sugars, essential fatty acids, and amino acids needed for optimal healing. Ideally, choose a product that contains protease, amylase, lipase, and disaccharidases like sucrose, maltose, and lactose.

You can also supplement with one or more of the following types of enzymes between meals on an empty stomach: bromelain, chymotrypsin, mucolase, papain, protease, superoxide dismutase (SOD), or trypsin or a single product that includes some or all these enzymes, as they can be helpful for allergies and asthma. Start with one capsule or tablet of your chosen enzyme on an empty stomach twenty minutes before or at least one hour after meals three times daily. You can gradually increase that amount to three capsules or tablets at a time three times daily or more with the guidance of a nutritional medicine practitioner experienced in systemic enzyme therapy.

Pick Pineapple Enzyme for Allergy Relief

Extracted from pineapple, when taken on an empty stomach the enzyme bromelain treats allergies, sinus inflammation and congestion, and other respiratory complaints because it acts as an anti-inflammatory on the tissues and helps reduce lung swelling. Here are some of bromelain's main functions:

- breaks down protein
- is anti-inflammatory
- improves digestion
- alleviates lung swelling
- speeds recovery
- reduces tissue swelling
- is good for sinusitis and respiratory disorders
- balances the immune system
- aids the body in identifying and destroying bacteria, including harmful ones that may reside in the gut
- helps alleviate allergies

Although pineapples naturally contain bromelain, the enzymes they contain normally work on digesting the fruit. Although you can certainly enjoy pineapple periodically (avoid eating too much of it or eating it too often, as it is extremely high in sugar, which can aggravate allergies), I usually suggest supplementation with this enzyme for allergy symptoms. Take one or two capsules containing 5000mcu each on an empty stomach three times daily. Because some enzymes can have blood-thinning effects, do not use them if you are taking blood-thinning drugs, are scheduled for surgery (and for at least a couple of weeks after surgery), or have another medical condition for which blood thinning could be a concern.

Enzyme Improves Asthma and Allergies

Serrapeptase, a natural enzyme, has been shown to aid asthma, allergies, and many other health conditions. It helps break down excessive mucus while alleviating the swelling of the sinuses.

Research by Dr. Nakamura and his colleagues at the Department of Respiratory Medicine at the Tokyo Metropolitan Hiroo General Hospital in Japan found that the enzyme dissolves excess mucus. He published his results in the journal *Respirology*, showing that serrapeptase assists the body to clear away excess mucus from the lungs in people with chronic conditions of the airways. He also found that serrapeptase reduced the amount of coughing linked to excessive mucus. The enzyme appears to work by restoring balance to an overactive immune system while at the same time thinning the mucus so it can be more effectively eliminated from the body.[2]

Serrapeptase may also be beneficial in treating other conditions involving inflammation. In a study published in the *Indian Journal of Pharmaceutical Sciences*, Drs. Viswanatha and Patil found that serrapeptase was more effective than aspirin at reducing inflammation in animals.[3] Additional research will indicate whether serrapeptase has the same beneficial effects in humans. But because the enzyme is safe for use, has very few side effects, and is highly therapeutic, it warrants consideration in the treatment of allergies.

Serrapeptase is also known as serratiopeptidase, serratia protease, or serrapeptidase and is available in many health food stores or online stores. It is best taken on an empty stomach. Choose a product containing twenty thousand serrapeptase or serratiopeptidase units. Take one capsule or tablet daily. Because some enzymes can have blood-thinning effects, do not use them if you are taking blood-thinning drugs, are scheduled for surgery (and for at least a couple of weeks after surgery), or have another medical condition for which blood thinning could be a concern. In extremely rare cases, some individuals have experienced an allergic skin reaction to serrapeptase. Discontinue use if you suspect an allergy to this supplement.

Papaya Enzymes Reduce Congestion

Papain is an enzyme that has been isolated from papaya fruit. It is a protein-digesting enzyme that has anti-inflammatory, anti-infectious, and diuretic properties. As such, it helps alleviate inflammation linked to sinus and nasal swelling. Additionally, it helps reduce infections in the gut that may play a role in allergies. It also helps address many of the symptoms of allergies, hay fever, and excessive catarrh buildup in the lungs, nasal passageways, or sinuses. It works on these root causes of allergies, so be patient: it may take some time with papain, like other enzymes, to see symptom relief. Papain is measured in papain units or in milligrams. Choose a product containing 250mg of papain. Take two capsules three times daily during allergy season. Papain and bromelain are often found in the same product. If that's the case, choose one containing 250mg of each. Take two capsules of this blended product three times daily.

Superoxide Dismutase (SOD) to Alleviate Allergies

According to the medical journal *Food and Function*, some naturally fermented foods like sauerkraut have been shown to boost levels of SOD, which is a powerful antioxidants that protects the body against free radical damage while also helping alleviate the symptoms of allergies.[4] SOD is one of the body's greatest weapons against illness, yet it requires sufficient amounts of zinc in the diet to work properly. You can eat more zinc-rich foods in your diet, including beets, beet greens, carrots, green leafy vegetables, nuts, onions, peas, pumpkin seeds, and most types of sprouts, to ensure your body can use SOD. Keep in mind that you should add zinc-rich foods to your diet but still take SOD supplements on an empty stomach. The zinc will get stored in your body for use later when you take SOD. SOD stores in the body tend to become diminished as we age, so supplementation is often helpful. Because this enzyme is so helpful in the treatment of many conditions, including allergies, it is worth considering as part of your allergy-relief program. Take two capsules three times daily.

Mucolase and Seaprose to Reduce Congestion

Little research has been done on mucolase or seaprose, but these enzymes are marketed for the purpose of dissolving mucus. Because they are both proteolytic enzymes—which means they digest protein—like other enzymes of this type, they should be effective at dissolving mucus, but they can be difficult to find. Follow package directions if you choose to use these products.

Broad-Spectrum Enzymes

The same enzyme supplement you may be taking with meals to improve digestion and nutrient absorption can also help treat allergies. In addition to taking the supplement with meals, you take it on an empty stomach. It also works against allergies because most digestive enzyme supplements contain a wide variety of enzymes, including amylase (which breaks down carbs), cellulase (which breaks down fiber or cellulose), chymotrypsin, trypsin, and protease (all of which break down proteins), among others. When these enzymes are taken on an empty stomach, there are no carbohydrates, fiber, or proteins to digest, so they begin working on inflammation, harmful infections, dissolving mucus, and other roles that boost the body's resilience against allergies.

I've included a chart of some of the best enzymes for allergies below. You'll find most of them in a broad-spectrum enzyme supplement. Take one to two capsules of your selected enzyme three times daily on an empty stomach.

Enzyme	Digestive Use	Function	Units
amylase	carbohydrate digesting	breaks down carbohydrates, including starch and glycogen reduces food cravings regulates histamine when taken on an empty stomach	dextrinizing units (DU) and Sandstedt Kneen Blish Units (SKB)
bromelain	protein digesting	breaks down protein is anti-inflammatory can be used in place of pepsin or trypsin with digestive difficulties is useful for lung swelling reduces tissue swelling	gelatin digesting units (GDU) and papain units (FCCPU)

Enzyme	Digestive Use	Function	Units
bromelain *(continued)*		is good for sinusitis and other respiratory concerns	
		balances the immune system	
		aids body in identifying and destroying harmful bacterial infections	
		helps allergies	
cellulase	carbohydrate digesting	breaks down cellulose in plant foods and chitin, a fiber found in the wall of yeasts (including *Candida albicans*, which is frequently involved in leaky gut syndrome)	cellulase units (CU)
		breaks down cell walls to free nutrients in fruits and vegetables	

Enzyme	Digestive Use	Function	Units
chymotrypsin	protein digesting	breaks down protein is anti-inflammatory reduces swelling helps liquefy mucus to aid secretion	milligrams (mg) or United States Pharmaco-peia (USP)
mucolase	protein digesting	breaks down mucus is helpful for congestion and sinus infections	mg and muco-lase units (MSU)
papain	protein digesting	breaks down protein is anti-inflammatory works sim-ilarly to chymotrypsin is a diuretic to alleviate swelling from the tissues is useful for allergies, hay fever, and catarrh treats infections	food chem-ical codex papain units (FCCPU)

Enzyme	Digestive Use	Function	Units
protease	protein digesting (used as a category of protein-digestive enzymes that includes bromelain, chymotrypsin, papain, pancreatin, and trypsin)	breaks down protein supports immune system functioning when taken on an empty stomach reduces inflammation	hemoglobin units in a tyrosine base (HUT)
seaprose	protein digesting	breaks down mucus aids congestion and sinus infections is a concentrated form of mucolase	mg
serratiopeptidase or serrapeptase or serrapeptidase	protein digesting	breaks down proteins is anti-inflammatory improves the immune system is used to treat sinusitis, allergies, and lung conditions	serratiopeptidase units (SU) or units

Enzyme	Digestive Use	Function	Units
superoxide dismutase (SOD)	protein digesting	is an antioxidant that protects the body against free radical damage is anti-inflammatory is one of the most potent antioxidant enzymes	
trypsin	protein digesting	breaks down proteins is anti-inflammatory aids hives, dermatitis, and eczema aids respiratory and throat conditions, including asthma and sinusitis	mg or USP

5

Natural Medicine That Works

WHEN IT COMES TO allergies, there are many essential nutrients, herbs, and other natural medicines that prevent and even reverse them. Most, if not all, natural medicines work differently from drugs. As you learned in chapter 1, drugs usually affect a single biochemical imbalance in the body, which in turn reduces symptoms but does not address the underlying cause or factors that are creating allergy symptoms in the first place. Whereas many natural medicines affect the body's biochemical processes to reduce symptoms, they also strengthen the body and its tissues, glands, and organs to correct the root of the problem.

Although many people—doctors included—used to believe that vitamins didn't have much of an effect on health, that idea has long been considered a medical myth. The reality is that nutrients impact every part of your body. Vitamins, minerals, phytonutrients (special plant nutrients), amino acids (the building blocks of protein), essential fats, carbs, enzymes (which we'll discuss in the next chapter), and other nutrients are needed in sufficient amounts to make healthy cells, tissues, glands, organs, and organ systems. Without adequate amounts of these essential nutrients, we cannot and will not experience the health we deserve.

VITAMINS: THE VITAL FACTOR FOR HEALTH

After years of extensive research, we now know that vitamins by definition are required for health. After all, the *Oxford Dictionary* defines *vitamin* as "any of a group of organic compounds which are *essential* for normal growth and nutrition and are required in small quantities in the diet because they cannot be synthesized by the body."[1] In other words, we cannot live without adequate vitamins, and we certainly cannot live a healthy, allergy-free life in their absence.

Every cell in your body needs particular vitamins to work properly. Without adequate vitamins, cellular functions begin to break down until there are potentially serious flaws in their workings. If this happens, the cells may even die off prematurely as the body tries to protect itself against possible damage. Alternatively, defective cells form the basis of tissues in the body that can result in disease or impaired function.

If even a single vitamin is deficient in the body, the results can be disastrous to our health. And as I can attest from having worked with thousands of people, one person's ideal amount of vitamins is another person's deficiency. That's because some people simply have higher needs for specific vitamins than others. The reality is that everyone is biochemically unique, and although we all need vitamins, minerals, and other nutrients for our survival and our optimal health, we need them in different quantities from the recommended dietary intakes put forth by government bodies. In the case of people vulnerable to allergies, it seems that a large proportion may have a vitamin C deficiency that food alone does not address.

Vitamin C: The Body's Super Stress Vitamin

I began conducting nutritional consultations almost twenty-five years ago. Over the years, I noticed that many people with allergy symptoms also had the symptoms of weakened adrenal glands. These two triangular-shaped glands that sit on top of the kidneys handle all our work, home, financial, relationship, and family stresses and much more. Yet most of us don't give them a second thought until we're allergic, exhausted, depressed, or experiencing other symptoms of adrenal stress—if we give them any thought at all.

With our increasingly hectic pace of life, an increasing number of people show signs of adrenal depletion. Some of the symptoms of depleted adrenal glands include the following:[2]

- asthma
- cold sweats or excessive perspiration
- depression
- dermatitis
- easily shaken up or heart pounds hard from unexpected noise
- emotional upsets cause complete exhaustion
- excessive neck, head, and shoulder tension
- excessive worrying
- eyes sensitive to bright lights
- hay fever
- nervousness
- skin rashes
- sneezing attacks
- unusual craving for salt

The adrenal glands must address everything that is a stressor to the body, whether we're aware of it or not. This onslaught of stresses can, over time, deplete the glands so they are overaggravated, underfunctioning, or alternating between the two states.

Some of the things that affect the adrenal glands include fear, anxiety, anger, financial pressures, toxic exposures (large or ongoing, like in our daily life), infections, inability to relax, insufficient sleep or rest, going to a job we don't like, excessive coffee or caffeine consumption, injuries, illness, marital problems, prescription or over-the-counter drug use, sugar consumption, poor eating habits, overexertion, cigarette smoking, illicit drug use, death of a family member, and even allergies. That's right: allergies can be, at least in part, the result of weakened adrenal glands, but ongoing allergy exposures can also serve to further aggravate and weaken the adrenal glands.

The adrenal glands use more vitamin C than any other organ or gland in the body. Vitamin C is essential to manufacture adrenal gland hormones. So when you've been chronically stressed in any of the previously mentioned ways, your adrenals may have depleted your vitamin C stores, which makes you more vulnerable to depleted adrenal glands and the conditions that accompany their overuse. And as you may have noticed from the list, there are many allergy-related symptoms linked to depleted adrenals.

In one study published in the medical journal *Food Science and Biotechnology*, researchers found that vitamin C was essential to manufacture two different hormones to help the body cope with stress and reduce the damaging effects of stress hormones.[3] Vitamin C has also been found to help the body effectively metabolize histamine so it is less likely to cause many of the symptoms linked to allergy symptoms.[4]

Vitamin C is primarily found in citrus fruits, berries, green and leafy vegetables, tomatoes, cabbage, cauliflower, broccoli, potatoes, sweet potatoes, cantaloupe, green peppers, and papaya, as well as most other fruits and vegetables to a lesser degree. However, the amount found in fruits and vegetables is insufficient to address allergy symptoms and potentially stressed adrenal glands and their higher needs during allergies.

For quick relief of allergy symptoms take 2000mg of vitamin C three times daily with at least two to three hours between doses, up to 10,000mg daily. This may seem like a lot of vitamin C, but when the body is under excessive stress its requirement for the nutrient skyrocket. Besides, it is water soluble, which means that your body will simply eliminate any excess vitamin it doesn't need at a particular time. In my experience, I have found that most adults will absorb about 2000mg in a single dose. And many people with allergies tolerate this dose several times a day. If you experience loose bowels, then you know you have exceeded the amount your body can tolerate in a single day. If that is the case, reduce the dose by 1000mg per day.

You may also notice that your vitamin C requirements change over time. For example, you may need 6000mg daily before you reach bowel tolerance, as it is called among health professionals. Several weeks later you may reach bowel tolerance after 2000mg of vitamin C. That is simply a sign that your adrenal glands have been rebuilding and have lower vitamin C needs.

Choose ascorbic acid over other forms of vitamin C, such as calcium ascorbate. In my experience, ascorbic acid is more effective at alleviating allergy symptoms.

FOURTEEN WAYS TO GIVE YOUR ADRENALS A BOOST

The adrenal glands are overworked and underappreciated thanks to our modern lifestyle. Fortunately it is easy to give them a boost, which goes a long way toward treating allergies too.

1. **Give the fast food a break.** Usually loaded with neurotoxins like monosodium glutamate (MSG), fast food can cause your body to be

in a constant state of stress after eating it and until the chemicals are detoxified from your system. Depending on the strength of your liver's detoxification systems, that can be anywhere from a few hours to several days.

2. Take a deep breath . . . and then take a few more. Research shows that even a few minutes of deep breathing can have an impact on the adrenal glands by reducing the stress hormones they secrete. Instead of jumping out of your seat during a traffic jam or other stressful spot, start breathing deeply.

3. Reduce your stress. I know this sounds impossible to many people, but the truth is that no one else is going to reduce your stress. Although life can be stressful sometimes, it's important to take some time daily to release stress. Go for a walk, stop and smell the roses (literally), give a loved one a hug, practice meditation, and get some rest.

4. Eat plenty of fresh fruit and vegetables. Chronic stress depletes nutrients. By eating a diet rich in nutrients from fresh fruit and vegetables, you'll give your body the vitamins, minerals, and phytonutrients to help it recover.

5. Reduce your caffeine intake. Caffeine stimulates the adrenal glands, only to cause an energy crash later on.

6. Try to get at least seven or eight hours of sleep at night. And if possible, don't wake to a blaring alarm clock, as the noise causes a flood of stress hormones to be released.

7. Practice the yoga posture Viparita Karani. For those of you who don't speak Sanskrit (myself included), that means, according to yoga expert Roger Cole, "legs up the wall, pelvis elevated on a bolster or folded blankets." He adds that "if the legs tire of being straight, bend the knees and cross the legs, with knees near the wall." According to Cole, "This pose stimulates baroreceptors (blood pressure sensors) in the neck and upper chest, triggering reflexes that reduce nerve input into the adrenal glands, slow the heart rate, slow the brain waves, relax blood vessels, and reduce the amount of norepinephrine circulating in the bloodstream."

8. Exercise regularly but don't overdo it. Exercise is a valuable release for pent-up stresses. Just know your limits and don't overexercise, as it can cause stress on the adrenals.

9. Take some extra vitamin B5, or pantothenic acid as its also known. Pantothenic acid is necessary for adrenal gland health. Although it is naturally present in the adrenal glands, it can become depleted as hormones are manufactured in response to stress. A common dose for adrenal fatigue is 1500mg but should always accompany a B-complex vitamin, as these nutrients work synergistically.

10. Avoid sugar and refined wheat products. They cause your blood sugar to fluctuate rapidly, which in turn cause your adrenals to overreact.

11. Eat some protein at every meal to help stabilize blood sugar and prevent strain on the adrenals. That doesn't necessarily mean meat. Some good vegetarian sources of protein include legumes (beans), nuts, seeds, avocado, and quinoa (a delicious whole grain).

12. Supplement with Siberian ginseng. Depending on how serious your adrenal stress may be, you may also benefit from herbal support *Eleutherococcus senticosus*, as it is also known. It works primarily on the pituitary gland in the brain to better regulate adrenal gland function. In adrenal fatigue, communication between the pituitary gland and the adrenals may be impaired. A typical dose of Siberian ginseng for the treatment of adrenal fatigue is 100 to 200mg daily.

13. Take a page from Ayurveda, the Indian form of natural medicine with a several-thousand-year-old history. Practitioners of Ayurvedic medicine recommend ashwagandha, or *Withania somnifera* as it is also known. Ashwagandha is a tonic for fatigue and exhaustion, memory loss, muscle weakness, and other symptoms of adrenal fatigue. It can normalize adrenal gland hormones. One to two teaspoons of an ashwagandha tincture daily is the commonly recommended dose. Always consult your physician prior to use.

14. Take some vitamin C. As I've also shown in this book, the adrenal glands need more vitamin C than any other organ or gland in the

> body. A typical dose to assist with adrenal stress is 500 to 2000mg
> or higher; however, higher doses may be necessary in some cases. If
> you use higher doses, it is best to take a maximum of 2000mg at a
> single time, wait a few hours, then take another dose.

Vitamin D

Most of us know that vitamin D is important to keep our immune system strong, but few people know that there are many other health benefits of getting enough of the sunshine vitamin. Vitamin D can help improve allergy symptoms, particularly by improving lung function. That's because a vitamin D deficiency is linked to a rapid decline in lung function, according to research published in the *American Journal of Respiratory and Critical Care Medicine*.[5] The researchers explored the relationship between vitamin D and smoking, lung function, and lung decline in 626 men. We all know that smoking harms lung function, but the researchers found that vitamin D had a protective effect on the lungs and reduced the rate of lung function decline, even among those with the highest risk of respiratory decline—smokers. Although the study focused on smokers because lung changes are easier to observe among these individuals, the lung improvements are sure to apply to nonsmoking allergy sufferers as well.

There are three primary sources of vitamin D: moderate sunlight exposure, food sources, and supplements. Tuna, salmon, and mackerel are the primary food sources of vitamin D, but beef liver and egg yolks also contain some. Because it is difficult to obtain all the vitamin D needed from sunlight or food, supplementation with D3 (also known as cholecalciferol, the type of vitamin D that has been used in most studies showcasing the vitamin's benefits), I also recommend supplementing with the vitamin to maintain a healthy respiratory system and reduce the impact of allergies. Although some sources suggest 800 IU daily for adults, most people actually need much higher amounts than that. I usually recommend 4000 IU daily for adults. Vitamin D is available in a liquid form that is readily absorbed under the tongue. Be sure to choose vitamin D3, not D2, which is actually a synthetic version of the nutrient.

Vitamin E for Respiratory Health

According to research published in the medical journal *Annals of Allergy, Asthma, and Immunology*, vitamin E supplementation reduces the severity of nasal symptoms linked to allergies. The study suggests that vitamin E supplementation may reduce the immune response at the root of allergies, not just the symptoms themselves, making this vitamin an excellent option to restore immune health and address nasal symptoms simultaneously.[6] Take 400 IU of a natural source vitamin E supplement, preferably taken as mixed tocopherols. This powerful antioxidant helps protect the lungs against toxins and their resulting damages. It is often part of a multivitamin, so you may not need to take additional vitamin E. Check your supplement to ensure you are getting adequate amounts. Vitamin E is actually a group of vitamins known as mixed tocopherols, which is the preferred type to take. Some products only contain alpha tocopherol, which is important, but it is better to take mixed tocopherols.

MINERALS THAT MANAGE ALLERGIES

Although there are many essential minerals that relax bronchial muscles prone to spasm in asthma sufferers, calcium and magnesium are especially important, as they work together to restore the mechanism involved with relaxing and contracting muscles. Adequate amounts of calcium ensure that muscles contract properly, whereas magnesium ensures that they relax properly. Both functions are necessary to ensure healthy breathing. I have found in my twenty-five years of practice that most asthmatics tend to be severely deficient in the mineral magnesium. To address this deficiency, take 250mg of both calcium and magnesium three to four times per day—three for men and four for women, for a total of 750 to 1000mg of each mineral daily. Cut back if you start to experience excessively loose bowel movements.

Take Quercetin to Quell Allergy Symptoms

Quercetin is an antioxidant, anti-inflammatory, and antihistamine phytonutrient, which simply means it is a nutrient that is derived from plant sources (*phyto* means "plant"). Quercetin has an excellent ability to reduce allergy symptoms and improve lung function.

This phytonutrient is best known for inhibiting the release of histamine, the chemical responsible for the uncomfortable symptoms of seasonal allergies. In a new study published in the medical journal *In Vivo*, researchers attempted to identify the mechanism by which quercetin works in people suffering from allergic rhinitis (allergy-caused nasal congestion). They found that quercetin significantly reduced the body's production of a particular protein known as periostin, which is a marker for airway inflammation.[7] Reducing this compound is an important part of addressing allergy symptoms for both short- and long-term success.

Both apples and onions are excellent sources of quercetin. Some studies show that people who eat a lot of apples have improved lung function and a reduced risk of lung conditions like asthma, which is likely due to their quercetin content. Although there are many good food sources of the nutrient, including apples, berries, cabbage, cauliflower, nuts (see note in chapter 2 on peanuts), and black, green, or white tea, allergy sufferers tend to need far more quercetin than diet alone offers.

Supplementing with the phytonutrient quercetin is also frequently helpful because, like vitamin C, it has antihistamine effects. Usually quercetin supplements also contain the enzyme bromelain, creating a powerful blend of allergy-reducing compounds. Take 400mg of quercetin twice daily. To quickly reduce allergy symptoms, take 2000mg of vitamin C alongside 400mg of quercetin.

As a bonus, many studies link quercetin intake to lower cholesterol levels, lower blood pressure (in those with high blood pressure), and a reduced risk of heart disease and many types of cancer, including prostate, colon, ovarian, breast, gastric, and cervical cancers. Taking quercetin for your allergies may give your overall health a boost too, which can't be said for drug options, with their long list of harmful side effects.

EGCG for Immune Support

Green tea contains a potent antioxidant known as epigallocatechin gallate (EGCG) that kills free radicals, which tend to be involved with allergies. Because it is a potent antioxidant, it can positively impact allergies on a cellular level by reducing both free radicals and the damage they cause as well as inflammation.

If you're not wild about the flavor, try a few different kinds. Try it iced or hot. Add some of the natural herb stevia to sweeten it if you want a sweeter drink. I wasn't crazy about green tea the first few times I tried it, but now, with a fresh squeeze of lemon and a few drops of stevia over ice—voilà! I love it! Green tea lemonade. *Mmmmm.* Even green tea haters love this drink.

Add one or two teaspoons of green tea leaves to a cup of boiled water, preferably in a tea strainer. Let steep for five minutes. Pour over ice if you prefer a cold beverage. I recommend three cups daily. And don't worry: it contains a lot less caffeine than coffee or black tea. Having said that, caffeine helps open the airways in the lungs, making it a valuable plant nutrient for asthma sufferers. However, it is best to consume no more than three cups of green tea daily, spread throughout the day. If you have insomnia or any sleep disorders, avoid drinking green tea after 3:00 p.m.

You can also supplement with additional EGCG. Most supplements do not contain caffeine, but check the label to be sure. This is an excellent way to obtain the lung-boosting, antioxidant, and anti-inflammatory effects of green tea and EGCG without the caffeine. For some people, caffeine makes them nervous, jittery, or anxious and is best avoided.

OTHER NATURAL ALLERGY-FIGHTING NUTRIENTS

A nutrient known as N-acetyl cysteine (sometimes called NAC) can be helpful in treating and healing allergies. This nutrient helps liquefy mucus in the bronchial tubes and is a potent antioxidant against free radical damage in the lungs. In a study published in the medical journal *Toxicology Sciences*, researchers found that NAC supplementation reduced the hyperreactivity of the lungs. Although the study explored the reactivity to diesel exhaust fumes, it is likely that this nutrient is helpful with other allergies to inhalants. The study dose was 600mg three times daily for six days. It may be beneficial to take this amount for a week and then to reduce the dose to 600mg daily after that. Prescribing a higher dose of certain nutrients at the beginning of the treatment is called a *loading dose*. It simply means that it helps get sufficient quantities into the bloodstream and tissues to ensure a faster reduction in symptoms; however, it is not a dose to continue with after that point. This approach is not suitable for all nutrients but seems to be helpful for NAC.

HERBAL MEDICINES THAT REALLY WORK

Many people are tempted to discount the effectiveness of herbal products, but they have helped humans survive on this planet for thousands of years, long before drug medicines became available in only the last century or two. Many herbs are surprisingly effective at reducing allergy symptoms and preventing future allergies. Some of my preferred herbal medicines include nettles, perilla, butterbur, and sea buckthorn.

Choose Nettles for Allergies

If you are a gardener, you are probably familiar with nettles because the plant's full name is stinging nettles, and it has little stingers along its stem that cause a prickling sensation when touched. I certainly remember my first encounter with this plant. Curtis, my husband of many years, dug up the grass at our first home together. A romantic, he wanted to create a stunning rose garden for me. He replaced the lawn with more than forty rose bushes and stone walkways. It was an artistic and stunningly beautiful creation that I still remember, even though we no longer live at this house. Every day, I would come home and no matter how stressful the events of the day had been, this loving gesture and beautiful garden would bring a smile to my face. One day, I was out weeding the garden and was feeling a bit lazy, so I didn't bother getting my gardening gloves. I grabbed a weed with the intention of yanking it out bare-handed, but the weed had other plans. I instantly recoiled as I felt a stinging sensation in my fingers. I had just become acquainted with stinging nettles and its survival tactics. I quickly learned to make the minimal effort to get my gardening gloves while weeding. But it was truly a miniscule price to pay for my husband's loving creation and beautiful garden. Soon afterward, I learned that this prickly plant had many healing properties worth considering, particularly when it comes to allergies.

Native Americans used stinging nettles for thousands of years to treat many health conditions, including allergies. Now science has proven what these wise people knew from experience: nettles are an effective allergy treatment. Unlike pharmaceuticals that cause heart problems or drowsiness, nettles do neither. In a study published in the medical journal *Phytotherapy Research*, Drs. Roschek, Fink, McMichael and Alberte at HerbalScience Group LLC, found that nettles worked on multiple levels to significantly reduce inflammation linked to allergies.[8]

Many markets now sell fresh nettles in the springtime. The fresh leaves are best cooked or made into an alcohol extract to nullify their stinging effects. It takes only about thirty seconds of cooking time to eliminate the sting when eating this highly nutritious plant. They can be added to soups and stews or sautéed like spinach or other green leafy vegetables. However, they are also conveniently available in the dried form for making tea, liquid tinctures to take as drops, or in capsule form if you want to skip the nettles-picking experience altogether. Medicinally, fresh nettles are far superior to dried ones, so it is worth donning a pair of thick gloves to harvest this healing plant. Avoid the use of nettles topically on open wounds or internally during pregnancy.

All these forms are excellent choices, but I have found liquid tinctures made with the fresh herb to be the best at alleviating allergy symptoms. You can make a tea using one heaping teaspoon of the dried herb per cup of boiled water, allowing it to steep for at least ten minutes, and then straining and drinking three cups daily for at least one month. Alternatively, take thirty drops of the tincture three times daily for at least one month. Follow package direction for products containing nettles capsules.

Perilla: The Little-Known Herb That Combats Allergies

Although it is tempting to run for the decongestants and antihistamines and lock yourself indoors during allergy season, Mother Nature offers help in the form of a little-known herb that can significantly improve most allergy symptoms. This mostly unknown herb, *Perilla frutescens*, is part of the mint family. Sometimes just called perilla, an extract from the plant's leaves have been found in many studies to be effective for the treatment of allergies, including nasal congestion, sinusitis, asthma linked to allergies, skin conditions, and eye irritation.

In one study published in *Experimental Biology and Medicine*, perilla and one of its active ingredients known as rosmarinic acid or rosmarinic extract were found to significantly ameliorate allergic inflammatory reactions such as nasal and sinus congestion as well as eye irritation.[9]

In another study published in *Phytotherapy Research*, Japanese scientists at the Department of Kampo Medicinal Sciences, Hokkaido College of Pharmacy, found that perilla was more effective than the drug tranilast, or the brand name Rizaben, which is used for allergies.[10]

And as if that wasn't convincing enough, still another study in the *International Journal of Molecular Medicine* found that perilla also alleviated allergic-related skin conditions.[11] Additionally, perilla has a beneficial effect on allergy-induced asthma symptoms, making it an excellent choice for asthmatics as well.

When the body's histamine levels remain high for long periods of time, as is the case with allergy sufferers, a person may also experience depression. Fortunately research in the *Chinese Journal of Natural Medicine* found that the essential oils naturally present in *Perilla frutescens* may also have an antidepressant effect.[12] It seems to work on multiple levels—reducing inflammation in the body, which most likely accounts for many of the herb's effects on allergies and depression, as well as boosting serotonin levels in the brain. Serotonin is a brain hormone, known as a neurotransmitter, which boosts our feelings of well-being.

The effective dose of perilla differs from product to product and depends on whether the seeds or leaves are used or whether the remedy is an extract of a specific compound or simply crushed dried leaves, among other factors. It is best to follow package directions for the product you select because there are both perilla leaves or perilla leaf extracts, which have a wide range in potency. A typical tincture dose is thirty drops three times daily. It is best to begin taking this herb about a month prior to your primary allergy season and throughout the season.

Butterbur Is Better than Allergy Medication

Butterbur, also known as *Petasites hybridus*, is a shrub that grows in wet, marshy areas in North America, Europe, and parts of Asia. The plant has been traditionally used for pain, headaches, fevers, and digestive problems. Multiple studies reveal that butterbur offers relief for allergy symptoms as well.

In a study published in the journal *Annals of Allergy, Asthma, and Immunology*, scientists at the British University of Exeter found that butterbur was as effective against allergy symptoms as a nonsedative allergy medication and more effective than the placebo used in the study.[13]

A study by Max Zeller Söhne, AG, in Romanshorn, Switzerland, and published in the journal *Phytotherapy Research* found that butterbur inhibited the allergic response and reduced allergic airway inflammation in animals exposed to allergens compared to the placebo, which had no effect on the animals.[14]

Another Swiss study comparing butterbur to the prescription allergy medication cetirizine, also known as Zyrtec, found that the effects of 8mg of butterbur four times a day are similar to those of cetirizine in patients with seasonal sinus and nasal congestion when evaluated blindly by patients and doctors. The scientists concluded that butterbur should be considered for treating seasonal allergies.[15]

The raw, unprocessed plant contains chemicals called pyrrolizidine alkaloids (PA) that can be harmful to humans, so butterbur products should clearly state that they are PA-free on the packaging. Unlike the drug cetirizine, butterbur does not have the following side effects: drowsiness, excessive tiredness, dry mouth, stomach pain, diarrhea, vomiting, difficulty breathing, or difficulty swallowing.

Supplement with Sea Buckthorn

An ancient Tibetan healing secret is finally being discovered in the West. For thousands of years Tibetans used a fruit that grows wild in the Himalayan Mountains as food and medicine to treat many serious health conditions ranging from breathing disorders to skin problems. Now science is proving that sea buckthorn is potent natural medicine.

Like many superfoods, sea buckthorn contains numerous powerful antioxidants that help the body deal with free radical damage (now linked to almost every illness and aging). But sea buckthorn doesn't stop there; it is also an excellent source of important omega-7s. And sea buckthorn is one of the best sources of this critical essential fat.

Sea buckthorn also contains more than 190 nutrients and phytonutrients, making it an extreme superfood. It has plentiful amounts of flavonoids, phytonutrients found in research to prevent cancer cells from multiplying while reducing pain and inflammation and contributing to weight loss in overweight individuals. The superfruit also contains plentiful amounts of the important healing enzyme superoxide dismutase (SOD)— actually, four times more than ginseng, another good source of SOD. SOD is important for maintaining strong respiratory health.

Asthma, chronic coughs, other breathing disorders, and allergy-related skin conditions are a few of the traditional uses for sea buckthorn, but it has also been shown to improve the health of eyes, mouth, and mucous membranes.

When it comes to skin conditions, it has been shown to be effective in a wide variety of ailments, including allergy-related skin problems like dermatitis and eczema. Many of its 190 nutrients are likely at work in these conditions, but its high amounts of omega-7s cause skin cell regeneration, minimizing wrinkling and the appearance of aging skin. Based on research published in the journal *Biochemical and Biophysical Research Communications*, scientists concluded that sea buckthorn could be used as a therapeutic agent against inflammatory skin diseases.[16]

If spring pollens aggravate asthmatic symptoms, you might want to supplement with sea buckthorn. Sea buckthorn has been used extensively in Traditional Chinese Medicine for lung conditions and asthma. Its use for asthma and chronic coughing are even recorded in the historic publication known as the *Tibetan and Mongolian Pharmacopoeia*.

As you learned in chapter 3, addressing gut health is also important when allergy-proofing your body. Sea buckthorn is a potent gut-health builder. Its gut-healing compounds combined with its natural anti-inflammatories make sea buckthorn an excellent choice for gastrointestinal (GI) complaints. The oil appears to provide a protective and healing coating to the stomach and GI tract, reducing the effects of harmful microbes like *E. coli* that could otherwise throw off the intestinal microbial balance and cause serious disease. The GI soothing and anti-inflammatory actions of sea buckthorn may seem irrelevant in a book about allergies, but as you learned in chapter 3, allergy elimination begins with gut health. It is important to kill any harmful microbes like *E. coli* and others that may reside in the intestines so they cannot inflame the intestines or perforate the gut wall. By reducing inflammation in the gut, beneficial microbes are more capable of thriving, and the combination, in turn, helps reduce inflammation elsewhere, such as the sinuses, nasal passageways, eyes, and lungs.

Hexane is used in the processing of most sea buckthorn on the market, even by many companies claiming that "vegetable oils" are used in the extraction of sea buckthorn's therapeutic compounds. Choose a reputable company that is committed to the highest standards of purity. There are many different sea buckthorn products, including berry oil and berry oil capsules, seed oil and seed oil capsules, and powder concentrates and capsules containing the concentrated powder as well as skincare products.

ELEVEN NATURAL LUNG-HEALING REMEDIES

From the greening up of nature in spring to the bountiful harvests and changing colors of trees in the fall, nature is a grand experience for most people, but for those suffering from allergies, asthma, or other breathing concerns, it is often a difficult time to breathe. Building up a strong respiratory system through the use of these eleven natural lung-healing remedies can immensely help in reducing allergy symptoms or the likelihood of experiencing allergies in the future. Of course, it's not necessary to use all these herbs; even just one or two will work fine. You can use them in a tea or tincture form, depending on preference and availability. Use one heaping teaspoon of herb per cup of boiled water, steeped for ten minutes for tea, drunk three times daily. Alternatively, use thirty drops (or about one teaspoon) of herbal tincture three times daily.

COLTSFOOT

Coltsfoot is an excellent herb for clearing out excess mucus from the lungs and bronchial tubes. In addition to clearing catarrh, it helps soothe coughs and protects and soothes mucous membranes. It has proven itself useful for asthma and other respiratory complaints. It combines well with horehound–the herb, not the candy.

ELECAMPANE

The root of the elecampane plant helps kill harmful bacteria in the gut, sinuses, and lungs, as well as lessens allergy-related coughs and expels excess mucus from the respiratory tract. It gradually alleviates any fever that might be present while battling infection and maximizing excretion of toxins through perspiration. If your allergy symptoms include a tickling cough or bronchitis, elecampane may be able to help. Because of its action on excess mucus and toxins in the respiratory tract, it is often helpful with asthma, bronchial asthma, and other respiratory conditions. In addition to the effects on the respiratory tract, it also helps a sluggish digestive system, thereby boosting gut health, which, as you know, is a factor in allergies.

EPHEDRA

There are many excellent herbal medicines that are valuable in the treatment of asthma. The plant ephedra is an excellent bronchodilator but can be difficult to obtain in some countries, where the plant's natural form is unavailable to health food stores thanks to regulators' overreaction to people abusing the plant in diet pills and supplements. Rather than insisting on warning labels similar to those used with the synthetic form known as pseudoephedrine, replete with many side effects not found in the natural herb, regulators simply made this amazing allergy remedy illegal for purchase in many places. By contrast, the synthetic version, pseudoephedrine, is readily available in over-the-counter allergy and cold and flu remedies but has a long list of side effects, as you learned in chapter 1. These synthetic versions are best avoided. I encourage people to write to your regulatory authorities and ask them to return this valuable remedy used for thousands of years to the marketplace. However, as with any type of medicine, not every remedy is right for all people. In some people, both the natural and synthetic forms of ephedra can cause heart palpitations, so avoid both the drug and the herb if you are prone to them. Also, it has a stimulating effect similar to caffeine, so don't take it in the evening.

HOREHOUND

Although you may prefer the candy from this bitter herb, it is the dried leaves that are best for their medicinal properties. They relax the muscles of the lungs while encouraging the clearing of excess mucus. Due to its antispasmodic properties, it is also good for bronchial spasms and coughs, which are common in allergy-induced asthma. Thanks to its highly bitter nature (which is why it is frequently blended with sugar), it is also good for digestive difficulties. The same bitter nature stimulates bile flow, thereby helping cleanse the digestive tract by initiating normal elimination from the intestines. Horehound combines well with coltsfoot, mullein, and lobelia to effectively clear the lungs.

LOBELIA

Lobelia is an excellent herb for lung concerns, coughs, respiratory infections, bronchial asthma, and excessive phlegm. It helps alleviate bronchial spasms, making it useful for asthmatics. It is an extremely strong herb and should therefore be used with caution. Rather than the dosage amounts listed above, it is best to follow package directions for lobelia. Do not exceed the recommended dose.

LICORICE ROOT

Licorice root is a natural anti-inflammatory herb that is beneficial in asthma. It also has antiviral effects and helps support the body's stress glands, the adrenals, which are often depleted in asthmatics. It can be taken in tea or tincture form. Add one teaspoon of the dried root to three cups of water, bring to a boil, and simmer over low heat, covered, for fifteen minutes. You can also buy licorice tea bags for convenience. To obtain sufficient therapeutic effects, be sure to buy tea bags that are only licorice root, not other herbs and flavors that dilute the medicinal effects of the tea. Drink one cup three times daily. Alternatively, take one teaspoon of the tincture two to three times daily.

LUNGWORT

Lungwort clears catarrh from the upper respiratory tract and bronchial tubes while helping soothe the mucous membranes and lessen coughs. It combines well with coltsfoot and horehound.

MARSHMALLOW

Marshmallow–the herb, not the fluffy white candy–is soothing to the mucous membranes of the lungs. It can be taken as a tea or tincture. For a tea, infuse one teaspoon of dried herb in one cup of water. Drink three cups daily.

MULLEIN

The leaves and flowers of the mullein plant soothe mucous membranes in the respiratory tract while clearing excess mucus. It lessens inflammation and pain, including within the nasal lining, throat, bronchial tubes, and digestive tract. It is helpful for allergy-induced coughs and bronchial inflammation.

PLEURISY ROOT

Pleurisy root is good for clearing out excess mucus from the lungs. It also has antispasmodic properties. If you are suffering from a large amount of mucus or catarrh buildup, pleurisy root works best when combined with coltsfoot. Combine a half to one teaspoon of dried herb per cup of water for a tea, drunk three times daily. Or take one-quarter to one-half teaspoon of tincture three times a day if you prefer.

SEA BUCKTHORN

Treating asthma, chronic coughs, other breathing disorders, and skin conditions are a few of the traditional uses for sea buckthorn, although the herb has found many more uses in recent times, including the treatment of cancer and skin conditions as well as for weight loss.

ESSENTIAL FATTY ACIDS AND FISH OILS FOR ALLERGY ALLEVIATION

Adequate amounts of essential fatty acids are needed to ensure lung, sinus, eye, and immune system health. Additionally, certain essential fatty acids like omega-3s act as a natural anti-inflammatory in the body to alleviate the low-grade inflammation underlying allergies and to address any inflammation involved in asthma. Omega-3s are the precursors of inflammation-regulating chemical messengers known as prostaglandins. Prostaglandins are made from omega-3 and omega-6 fatty acids. Both types of essential fatty acids are required, but the ratio is what matters most, as you learned in chapter 2. The vast majority of the population is deficient in omega-3 fatty acids, which can cause inflammation to go unchecked in the body, resulting in any number of health issues, including allergies or asthma. Omega-3 fatty acids are primarily found in the oils of cold-water fish, such as salmon, mackerel, herring, sardines, and anchovies, as well as nuts and seeds like flax, hemp, and walnut.

Thanks to low-fat diet fads, many people incorrectly believe that fat is not essential to the health of our bodies. But dietary fats are broken down into components known as fatty acids, which are the building blocks of fatty components of the body, including the respiratory and immune systems, both of which are involved in regulating allergies in the body.

By supplementing with fish oils you can help quickly restore a healthy balance of omega-3 fatty acids in your body. Fish oils are among the best supplements for reducing inflammation thanks to two active essential fatty acids known as eicosapentanoic acid (EPA) and docosohexanoic acid (DHA). These two types of omega-3s convert in the body into hormone-like substances that decrease inflammation.

Some people take fish oils and expect immediate symptom relief, but the fatty acids found in fish oil go to work to heal the underlying issues in the body, thereby reducing inflammation, which in turn will help reduce symptoms over a longer period of time. Although it is possible to obtain immediate results, most people need to continue supplementing with fish oil supplements for a few months to obtain their full benefit.

Once your symptoms level off, you may be able to reduce your dosage of fish oils or obtain your fish oils from eating fatty fish several times a week. I prefer a supplement combination of DHA and EPA, as both of these fats are needed to reduce inflammation in the body. There's also great news for people who are deficient in these nutrients: people who are deficient of omega-3 fatty acids absorb twice as many fatty acids once they start supplementing with them, compared with people who already have sufficient amounts.

Take two capsules of 1000mg of fish oils daily, for a total of 2000mg per day. For best results, each capsule should contain at least 180mg of EPA and 120mg of DHA. They are best taken with food to increase absorption and to reduce the fishy aftertaste some people experience. If you take them with food and still have gas and a fishy aftertaste, you may be deficient in the enzyme lipase that is needed to digest fats. If so, simply take a full-spectrum digestive enzyme formula that contains lipase along with your fish oil or DHA-EPA supplement.

Because some sources of fish have become polluted, look for a fish oil supplement or a DHA and EPA supplement that is confirmed by third-party laboratory results to be uncontaminated with mercury and other pollutants. Although I am not aware of any fish oil supplements being made from genetically modified fish, as of the writing of this book, genetically modified salmon was approved for sale in some countries, so keep in mind that GMOs could become a concern in fish oil supplements in the future.

6

Allergy Relief at
Your Fingertips

IMAGINE BEING STRUCK BY an arrow in an ancient battle and recovering from the wound only to discover that your life-long breathing difficulties and chest pains also disappeared. That is the legend behind the formation of acupuncture and its related needle-free therapy, acupressure. Wounded soldiers were believed to have experienced the sudden healing of pre-battle afflictions alongside the recovery of the arrow wound. Although the story may have been embellished, there is good reason that acupuncture and acupressure have stood the test of time for more than five thousand years: it works. And when it comes to allergies, it is a highly effective therapy that, when performed regularly, can help relieve pain and improve your body's healing ability. Hundreds of studies now demonstrate the effectiveness of acupuncture for healing many conditions, including in the treatment of nasal and sinus congestion, asthma, coughing, watery and irritated eyes, and other allergy symptoms.

Even the World Health Organization endorses acupuncture by publishing a list of dozens of illnesses that acupuncture effectively treats, including sinusitis, rhinitis (nasal congestion), asthma, conjunctivitis (eye inflammation), and headaches and migraines, which can all be linked to allergies. But you don't need needles to benefit from this remarkable healing therapy.

Traditional Chinese Medicine includes many points on the body that can be massaged to support healing from common allergies and other common health conditions. You can easily massage these points on your own hands or body or ask a partner to massage the points on your hands or body, depending on the point locations. These healing points are also called acupoints. Numerous scientific studies have shown the existence of these acupoints, which are located along invisible energy lines called *meridians* or *channels* that connect to various organs and systems in the body. When pressed or massaged, these points can induce therapeutic functions that are specific to each point, from reducing watery and itchy eyes to alleviating sinus and lung congestion.

Meridians are similar to rivers. If a tree falls in a river, it may disrupt the flow of water through the river and may even affect any tributaries that flow from the river. A blockage along the meridian is similar to a tree that falls in the water: it may disrupt the proper flow of energy throughout the body. When blockages occur, we experience many possible symptoms ranging from fatigue to pain. If the blockages continue over time, we experience any number of possible illnesses, including allergies. Using finger pressure at the points where the blockages occur helps them to disperse, thereby allowing the free flow of energy along the meridians again. When energy flows smoothly, we experience freedom from negative symptoms and better overall health.

Some of the benefits of using acupressure include:

- It is free.
- It is easy to do.
- It can be done anywhere.
- There are no harmful side effects.

There are many reasons why acupuncture and acupressure work. Study after study shows that these traditional therapies, which span thousands of years of use and success, work. That's probably why they have stood the test of time. But it's not important to understand all the theory, art, and science behind acupressure to put it to work for you.

HOW TO ALLEVIATE ALLERGIES WITH ACUPRESSURE

Based on the same premise as acupuncture, acupressure uses finger pressure instead of needles to unblock the flow of energy that runs along the meridians. Using simple acupressure techniques combined with the dietary and lifestyle suggestions in this book, you can heal from allergies.

Although there are hundreds of acupressure points on the body, it is not essential to know all the points to benefit from them. Some points are found in the area of where you experience allergy symptoms, whereas others are not. Although proponents of acupressure often espouse specific approaches to pressing or rubbing the points, you can get great results from doing what feels right for you and not getting caught up in theory. Most people find that holding the points firmly works well for them; some points work best with vigorous massage. Feel free to do what feels best for you. Where appropriate, I've specified those points that tend to be most effective with vigorous massage.

Please be patient. It may take some time while holding or massaging the points for the best results. And you might not experience it immediately afterward either. But with consistent use daily, the effort will be worth it. If you cannot press the points yourself, you might want to enlist the help of someone else to do it for you. If that's not possible, there are some good devices on the market that can help. Two of the most common are small, handheld low-level lasers, such as the Beurer laser, which is about one hundred dollars and is quite effective. There are also many electro-stimulation devices that use low levels of electricity to stimulate the acupoints, such as the Pointer Plus, which is also around one hundred dollars. Whereas they use light or electricity on the acupoints, they have a similar effect to acupressure.

Avoid using massage oils or lotions when rubbing the points, as these will typically make your skin too slippery to hold the point for any length of time. Most people find that holding the point for at least a few minutes is best.

You can be fully clothed while doing acupressure, making it easy to do anywhere. Some of the points are easily accessible and allow you to rub them in line at the grocery store, on a bus ride or in the car (as a passenger, of course), or while watching television. If it is difficult for you to use your thumb or fingers to hold the points, you can also use your knuckle.

Avoid getting stressed out over whether you are finding the point precisely. Frequently there will be some discomfort at the site of the point, whereas other times there will not be any noticeable sensation.

Most of the points are located on both sides of the body, with the exception of points along two channels known as the Du and Ren channels and the occasional Extra point. I'll explain more about these points momentarily. Most allergy symptoms, such as nasal congestion or watery eyes, tend to occur on both sides of the body; however, if only one sinus or eye is affected, hold the acupoints on the side of the body that you experience symptoms. For example, if you have discomfort and congestion in your left sinus only, hold the points on the left side of your body. If you experience discomfort on both sides of your body, which is the case for most people, hold the points on both sides for best results. If you cannot reach the point on the inflamed or aggravated side of the body, holding the point on the opposite side will still produce healing results and a lessening of symptoms.

I included the names of the point and the organ meridian they are linked to for your information; however, it is not essential knowledge to effect results. Afterward, I have described the location in words, but you can also look at the illustrations to find the area to massage. A general rule of thumb is that if you find a point on your body that feels sore, gently apply pressure or massage it—you may have discovered an energy blockage. Rubbing the area will help disperse any blockages you might have. Don't be overly aggressive while rubbing the area or you may cause bruising.

Don't be surprised if some of the points I am recommending are not even close to the location of your symptoms like sinus congestion or a runny nose. In Chinese medicine, some of the best healing points are located somewhere totally different on the body. Yet they are proven to be effective for healing and have been in use for thousands of years.

If you are pregnant, you should avoid using some points—namely, LI 4. Although there are other points to avoid during pregnancy, they are not among those described below. Avoid using acupressure during the first and last trimester of pregnancy as well. Pregnant or not, if you are uncertain whether to use acupressure or whether acupressure will negatively impact your health, please consult a qualified acupuncturist first.

Acupressure may look difficult at first, but it is really quite simple. With practice, you will find that it becomes easier. Soon you will be reaching for the exact points at the first sign of allergy symptoms. Even when your allergy symptoms subside, continue to use these points regularly to help maintain health and to reduce the frequency and severity of allergy symptoms. I urge you to take the initial time to become familiar with using acupressure, as it is such a powerful healing modality. You will find that it quickly becomes second nature and that soon you won't need to look at the illustrations and will instead start pressing the points at the slightest sign of allergy symptoms.

Below you will find some of the best points to deal with various allergy symptoms, from nasal and sinus congestion to itchy and watery eyes and even asthma. Because there is so much overlap between the points used for each of these symptoms, I have instead put them all together for a single thorough acupressure treatment for allergies. Additionally, because asthma can be such a serious and even life-threatening condition, I have added specific points for allergy-induced asthma. If you are suffering from allergy-induced asthma, I encourage you to use the acupoints recommended for both allergies and asthma.

I have listed the points using their traditional nomenclature in Chinese medicine, but don't be overly concerned that there are points called *Kidney 3* or *Stomach 41* or other seemingly unrelated names. And yes, if you have kidney or stomach concerns, you may find that using these points for your allergies also inadvertently improves your symptoms of these seemingly unrelated conditions. In Chinese medicine, they are frequently linked.

The key to effective acupressure is regularity. It is not adequate to do self-acupressure once per week; daily treatments are ideal. Two to three times daily is even better. Try to take the ten minutes or so per day to improve your pain and healing with this powerful modality. Massage as many of the following points as you can as a treatment for allergy symptoms and even when your symptoms are not too bad. Doing so can significantly reduce the frequency and severity of allergies over time.

> *Du 20 (Du channel).* The Du channel is one of the two main channels to supply energy to all the other meridians. It runs along the spine and over the head to the lips. Du 20 is arguably the most powerful point on the body and is located on the top of the head, about two-thirds of the way

to the back of the head, directly in the middle if you drew an imaginary line from the chin over the nose, between the eyes and over the head. It is found in a slightly soft spot that is sometimes tender to touch.

Lu 1 (lung meridian) is located on the front of the chest where it meets the shoulder joint.

Lu 7 (lung meridian) is located on the inside of the wrist approximately one inch above the wrist line toward the outer thumb edge.

Lu 9 (lung meridian) is located on the inside of the wrist crease toward the thumb-side edge of the wrist.

LI 4 (large intestine meridian) is located at the top of the crease when you push your thumb against your forefinger.

LI 19 (large intestine meridian) is located on the upper lip immediately below the nostrils.

LI 20 (large intestine meridian) is located just beside the outer edge of the nostrils.

Sp 10 (spleen meridian) is located on the upper leg about an inch above the top border of the kneecap toward the inside of the leg. Although it may seem completely unrelated to allergies, Sp 10 is actually one of the best points to alleviate allergy symptoms, particularly when it is vigorously massaged.

GB 21 (gall bladder meridian) is located on the top of the shoulder about halfway between the outer edge of the shoulder joint and the neck.

Ex 1 (Extra point 1) is located midway between the inner edges of the eyebrows. This point is good for allergy-induced headaches, nasal congestion, and issues with the eyes.

ALLERGY-INDUCED ASTHMA

If seasonal allergies have aggravated asthma symptoms and/or other lung concerns, emphasize the following points. Of course, you can still use the other allergy points mentioned above. And if you are suffering from an acute asthma attack, be sure to seek appropriate medical attention.

Du 20 (Du channel). The Du channel is one of the two main channels to supply energy to all the other meridians. It runs along the spine and over the head to the lips. Du 20 is arguably the most powerful point on the body and is located on the top of the head about two-thirds of the way to the back of the head, directly in the middle if you drew an imaginary line from the chin over the nose, between the eyes and over the head. It is found in a slightly soft spot that is sometimes tender to touch.

Ren 17 (Ren channel). The Ren channel is the other of the two main channels that supply energy to all the other meridians. It runs from the base of the lips along the front of the body to the base of the spinal column. This point is found in the middle of the chest, on the ribcage, at the midpoint between the nipples.

Ren 22 (Ren channel). This point is found on the Ren channel along the midline of the front of the body in the notch in the sternum between the collar bones.

Lu 1 (lung meridian) is located on the front of the chest where it meets the shoulder joint.

Lu 6 (lung meridian) is located on the inside of the arm where the lighter skin meets the darker skin, about four finger widths below the elbow crease.

Lu 7 (lung meridian) is located on the inside of the wrist approximately one inch above the wrist line toward the outer thumb edge.

Lu 9 (lung meridian) is located on the inside of the wrist crease toward the thumb-side edge of the wrist.

7

Medical Aromatherapy
to Ease Allergies

AROMATHERAPY 101

BATH AND BEAUTY COMPANIES have led most people to believe that aromatherapy is beneficial for relaxation, skin care, and bathing. Although it definitely helps in these regards, medical aromatherapy—a scientific approach to aromatherapy that uses the potent natural chemical constituents found in key essential oils—has been proven to dramatically reduce pain and inflammation and to aid healing and even restore normal pain signals to the brain, a common problem in longtime arthritis sufferers.

Aromatherapy is the therapeutic use of natural oils from flowers, plants, trees, resins, and other elements in nature that have healing properties. Aromatherapy is as old as nature itself, but humans have been using the art and science of aromatherapy therapeutically for at least six thousand years. There is plenty of archaeological evidence to suggest that aromatherapy oils were regularly used in the ancient temples of Egypt, Greece, and Rome. Our ancient ancestors must have observed that the scents of flowers, trees, and other plants had an impact on their stress levels, anxiety, sleep, mood, pain, and more.

Not only is aromatherapy one of the most powerful and fast-acting medical therapies available; it can also be a supremely enjoyable experience. Fragrant scented oils absorb through the skin into the bloodstream during massage. Alternatively, they diffuse into the air, where they are inhaled through our nose, giving many of the molecules direct access to the brain. Thanks to our drug-, surgery-, and radiation-based system of medicine, most of us have been led to believe that medicine must be harsh to be effective; aromatherapy seems too pleasurable to be effective medicine, but because it quickly gains access to the blood and brain, impressive results are common and fast acting.

When you smell essential oils—the oil-based potent plant extracts—you're actually breathing in the molecules of essential oils wafting in the air, which send signals directly from the cells in the nose to the brain. The brain then sends messages back to the body depending on the original message sent to the brain, which vary depending on the scent (or scents) and the chemical constituents they contain. These signals then act accordingly, to either reduce inflammation, relax the nervous system, boost mood enhancers, increase energy, reduce pain, or some other action depending on the initial chemical constituents detected in the essential oil.

Over the last several decades, research at some of the world's leading universities on the effects of essential oils on pain, inflammation, infection, depression, dementia, and many other symptoms and have found them effective for many of the ills we experience.

Essential oils have unique therapeutic traits and can contain more than one hundred chemical constituents, each of which produces unique effects in the body. Even the same plant grown in different conditions can result in different chemical constituents and, therefore, different therapeutic effects. Additionally, each plant can produce more than one type of oil; for example, there are two types of essential oils derived from the orange tree: neroli oil from the blossoms and orange oil from the peel of the oranges. But it isn't necessary to understand the complex chemistry of the plants and their oils to reap the rewards they offer.

Oils can be divided into one of three main classifications based on their general properties: uplifting, balancing, or calming. Uplifting oils tend to boost mood and energy levels, balancing oils tend to regulate imbalanced hormones and brain messengers known as neurotransmitters, which have a balancing effect on the body. Calming oils tend to relax the nervous system, and some even have sedative properties to improve sleep quality. Momentarily I'll share some of the most effective antipain and anti-inflammatory essential oils along with how to benefit from them.

CHOOSING ESSENTIAL OILS

It is important to choose high-quality oils because the therapeutic effects are greatly diminished in lesser oils. Although there are many types of oils in the marketplace, few are produced to maintain the integrity of the plant. Avoid oils from some of the large bath and body product shops, as these oils tend to be extremely low grade, are frequently diluted with other cheaper oils, and often contain synthetic ingredients. Also, avoid oils that are labeled "fragrance" oils, "perfume" oils, or "natural-like" oils, as they're usually synthetic chemicals that offer no therapeutic value whatsoever. Many of these synthetic oils are also hidden in perfumes, scented air "fresheners," laundry soaps, fabric softeners, and many other consumer products, which we'll discuss in greater detail in chapter 8. Even grocery bags are frequently scented with these toxic substances and are best avoided in favor of unscented varieties.

Instead choose undiluted pure essential oils that have been wild crafted or contain organic ingredients. Keep in mind that some claim their products are "pure" or "natural," but these terms mean nothing, as there are no quality-control standards required to be met to make these claims. Some companies also claim their products are "therapeutic grade," but similar to the terms pure and natural, this claim holds little if any merit at all.

Because essential oils are highly concentrated, a little goes a long way. It is best to use them as directed. Avoid taking the essential oils internally. Although some companies espouse this practice, it is best left to those with advanced medical aroma-therapy knowledge, as some oils can be toxic when used inter-nally. Also avoid contact with the delicate mucous membranes of the eyes and mouth. It's always best to dilute an essential oil and conduct a test patch on the inner wrist. Some essential oils can cause irritation to the skin when used undiluted, so only use oils that specify that using them in this manner is acceptable. For example, thyme oil is highly concentrated and can be irritating to the skin when it is undiluted, but many people can tolerate it by diluting a drop in a teaspoon of carrier oil like grapeseed, sweet almond, or apricot kernel oil and applying it to their skin. Additionally, the oil penetrates the skin and is absorbed into the bloodstream where it can help reduce allergy symptoms and stop the immune system from overworking.

Some oils can cause photosensitivity, which means they can make your skin more sensitive to the sun. These oils typically include citrus and bergamot oils. Avoid using these oils within a few hours of direct sun exposure on your skin or if you know you'll be spending a significant amount of time outdoors on a sunny day. The effect typically wears off within a few hours, so you can still benefit from these oils on other days or in the evenings after you've come indoors.

Essential oils are sold in small bottles and may seem expensive for their size, but keep in mind that you'll be using minute amounts of these oils at a time, so they'll last for long periods. Although essential oils should be undiluted when they are sold, you should dilute them in a carrier oil such as sweet almond, apricot kernel, grapeseed, avocado, or hazelnut oil to apply them to your skin. You can apply the oil blend directly on the affected area such as sinuses or just under the nose to alleviate congestion. Because the skin on the face tends to be more sensitive than other skin on our body, it is important to adequately dilute any essential oils used for this purpose. You can find both essential oils and carrier oils from reputable suppliers like Mountain Rose Herbals (see the Resources section for more information).

Although you can use diffusers that scent a room with the desired oils, it is best to avoid aromatherapy oil burners, as they alter the chemical structure of molecules in the essential oils, rendering them less therapeutic. Additionally, they tend to smoke, which only further aggravates sinus and nasal congestion, asthma, and difficulty breathing.

A QUICK GUIDE TO SELECTING ESSENTIAL OILS FOR ALLERGIES

There are many essential oils that are effective for allergy symptoms and for alleviating sinus congestion, sneezing, respiratory problems, and so forth. The following list is not exhaustive but includes oils that are readily available and highly effective for allergies. I've included safety information for each of the recommended oils. Remember that it is not necessary to use all the oils; actually, it is preferable that you stick with one or a blend of one to three oils at a time. I've included the Latin names of the preferred varieties of each essential oil to help ensure that you obtain the correct oils and avoid using any varieties that may lack therapeutic properties or, worse, be harmful.

Best Oils for Allergies

Some of my favorite essential oils for allergies include:

Blue Tansy, also known as *Moroccan chamomile* (*Tanacetum annuum*), contains a unique compound known as chamazulene that has natural antiallergic and antihistamine properties, thereby reducing allergy symptoms while also preventing more allergic reactions.

Eucalyptus (*Eucalyptus radiata* and *Eucalyptus globulus*). Both types are excellent expectorants that help clear sinus and lung congestion. Eucalyptus is highly effective at alleviating stuffed nasal passageways. Place a few drops on a tissue and inhale deeply for five to ten minutes. Alternatively, simply placing this one oil in an aromatherapy diffuser can help alleviate the congestion of allergies. Some people can handle one drop of this oil "neat," which means undiluted on the skin. Eucalyptus oil is especially helpful when used directly on the skin beneath the nose so you breathe it in with every breath. Do a seventy-two-hour test patch on the inside of your wrist to assess sensitivity to this oil used neat on your skin.

Khella (*Ammi visnaga*). This essential oil has antispasmodic and bronchodilating properties, which means it helps open up the passageways in the lungs and relieves the spasms in the smooth muscle tissue of the bronchi, the main passageways into the lungs.

Peppermint (*Mentha piperita*) works as a natural decongestant to alleviate nasal and sinus congestion. Unlike most essential oils, peppermint can be used neat to help reduce the congestion and headaches that often accompany allergies. A little goes a long way, as this oil leaves an intensely cooling sensation to the skin. Use only one drop under your nose to help sinuses drain. Be sure to conduct a seventy-two-hour test patch on the inside of your wrist to determine whether you have any skin sensitivity to it before using this oil neat on your face. Wash your hands immediately and avoid eye contact.

Tarragon (Artemesia dracunculus) has antiallergic properties that halt, reduce, and treat allergic reactions.

Thyme (Thymus satureioides and *Thymus vulgarus).* Both of these types of thyme balance your immune system to prevent overworking as it does in the case in allergies.

Keep in mind that it's not necessary to use all these oils to benefit from them. Choose the ones that you are able to find and that fit within your price range. Additionally, other than peppermint and eucalyptus, do not use the oils undiluted; they need to be diluted in a carrier oil to prevent skin or respiratory reactions and to obtain the best results. Although it has become common for some companies to recommend use of their essential oils for internal use, I do not advise this practice unless you are working with a highly trained medical aromatherapist.

Allergy-Proof Essential Oil Blend

20 drops blue tansy/Moroccan chamomile oil
   (*Tanacetum annuum)*
20 drops khella oil (*Ammi visnaga)*
20 drops peppermint oil (*Mentha piperita)*
20 drops tarragon oil (*Artemesia dracunculus)*
20 drops thyme oil (*Thymus satureioides* and
   Thymus vulgarus)

Add all the above essential oils to a small bottle (approximately 10mL) that has a lid. Place the lid on the bottle and tighten. Gently roll the jar of oil between your palms to evenly disperse the essential oils. Do not shake the oil as it will bring oxygen into the oil, which will accelerate the degradation of the oil.

Use a few drops of this oil in an aromatherapy nebulizer, which is a small gadget you can plug in and it will disperse microscopic droplets of the essential oils into the air. Use for ten to twenty minutes three times a day in whichever room you'll be in (bedroom, living room, office, etc.). Breathe deeply.

This oil is too concentrated for use on the skin; however, most people can tolerate one drop of this oil rubbed into the palms of their hands once or twice a day. In other words, place one drop of the oil onto the palm of one hand and rub your palms together to disperse the oil onto both palms. The oils readily absorb into the bloodstream for quick allergy and asthma improvements. It normally takes about twenty minutes to begin working; however, ideally you should begin this treatment about two months prior to allergy season for the best results. Do not use this oil undiluted on any other part of your body. Discontinue using it neat if the skin on your palms becomes irritated.

BEST OILS FOR ASTHMA

Some of my favorite oils that help reduce asthma symptoms include:

> *Black Spruce* (*Picea mariana*). In addition to having both anti-inflammatory and antispasmodic properties that aid asthma sufferers, this oil has natural compounds that strengthen and heal the adrenal glands.
>
> *Blue Tansy*, also known as *Moroccan chamomile* (*Tanacetum annuum*), contains chamazulene that has natural antiallergic and antihistamine properties that reduce allergy-induced asthma attacks.

Hyssop Decumbens (*Hyssopus off. var. decumbens*) is an excellent anti-inflammatory and a natural expectorant that helps eliminate mucus from the lungs.

Khella (*Ammi visnaga*). This essential oil has antispasmodic and bronchodilating properties, which means it helps open up the passageways in the lungs and relieves the spasms in the smooth muscle tissue of the bronchi, the main passageways into the lungs.

Scotch Pine (*Pinus sylvestris*) strengthens the adrenal glands to help heal asthma and reduce the effects of stress.

Star Anise (*Illicium verum*) has antispasmodic effects that prevent and treat spasms in the lungs linked to asthma.

Tarragon (*Artemesia dracunculus*). In addition to this oil's antiallergic properties, it also has antispasmodic effects on the lungs to prevent and treat the spasms often linked to asthma.

Keep in mind that it's not necessary to use all these oils. Choose the ones that you are able to find and that fit within your price range. Additionally, do not use the oils undiluted; they need to be diluted in a carrier oil to prevent skin or respiratory reactions and to obtain the best results. Although it has become common for some companies to recommend use of their essential oils for internal use, I do not advise this practice unless you are working with a highly trained medical aromatherapist.

Asthma Essential Oil Blend

20 drops black spruce oil (*Picea mariana*)
20 drops blue tansy/Moroccan chamomile oil
(*Tanacetum annuum*)
20 drops khella oil (*Ammi visnaga*)
20 drops hyssop decumbens oil (*Hyssopus off. var. decumbens*)

20 drops tarragon oil (*Artemesia dracunculus*)
20 drops Scotch pine oil (*Pinus sylvestris*)
20 drops star anise oil (*Illicium verum*)

Add all the above essential oils to a small bottle (approximately 10mL) that has a lid. Place the lid on the bottle and tighten. Gently roll the jar of oil between your palms to evenly disperse the essential oils. Do not shake the oil, as it will bring oxygen into the oil, which will accelerate the degradation of the oil.

Use a few drops of this oil in an aromatherapy nebulizer, which is a small gadget you can plug in and it will disperse microscopic droplets of the essential oils into the air. Use for ten to twenty minutes three times a day in whichever room you'll be in (bedroom, living room, office, etc.). Breathe deeply.

This oil is too concentrated for use on the skin; however, most people can tolerate one drop of this oil rubbed into the palms of their hands once or twice a day. In other words, place one drop of the oil onto the palm of one hand and rub your palms together to disperse the oil onto both palms. The oils readily absorb into the bloodstream for quick allergy and asthma symptom improvements. It normally takes about twenty minutes to begin working. Do not use this oil undiluted on any other part of your body. Discontinue using it neat if the skin on your palms becomes irritated.

If you are having an asthma attack, you can use this oil on your palms to help reduce wheezing and spasms in the lungs and improve your ability to breathe; however, do not use it as a replacement for your asthma inhaler or medical intervention.

How to Make Your Own Antiallergy Massage Oil

You can make your own aromatherapy oil to boost your health and to balance your immune system while alleviating symptoms.

Here's what you'll need:

¾ cup of a carrier oil (sweet almond, apricot kernel, grapeseed, liquefied coconut, or other oil of your choice)

30 drops of your choice of the essential oils for allergies as listed above, or use the Allergy-Proof Essential Oil Blend if you can (e.g., you might select thyme, eucalyptus, and peppermint)

Small to medium-sized glass bottle or jar with a lid to store the finished oil

Pour the carrier oil into the glass jar. Add the essential oils of your choice. Tightly close the bottle or jar with a lid. Gently roll the jar of oil between your palms to disperse the essential oils. Do not shake the oil, as it will bring oxygen into the oil, which will accelerate the degradation of the oil.

Massage the oil onto your skin, especially over the chest area.

8

More Natural Approaches to Allergy-Proof Your Body

WHEN IT COMES TO allergies, one of the most critical steps to take is to eliminate the harmful chemicals that can damage your respiratory and immune systems. Sadly, the home we consider our sanctuary is often full of toxic chemicals that cause or aggravate allergies and allergy-induced asthma. From personal-care products to laundry soaps and fabric softeners, many of the products we use daily should be replaced with natural, healthier options. This is especially true for allergy sufferers. Let's take a look at some of the worst culprits.

THE SHOCKING TRUTH ABOUT AIR FRESHENERS

It may seem obvious to state that we need air to breathe properly and to live a healthy life. But so few people give any consideration to the air they breathe—the same air that may be contributing to the respiratory and sinus issues linked to allergies. No book on allergies would be complete without a discussion of the harmful things we are doing to our air quality, starting with so-called air fresheners.

Before you spray Febreze, plug in a Glade PlugIn, light a scented candle, or use some so-called air freshening wick, mist, aerosol, or other car or room deodorizer, think twice. You'll be shocked to learn their ingredients and the harmful effects they can cause. That "Cleansing Rain," "Summer Breeze," "Fresh Country," "Cool Morning Air," or "Berry Burst" might be aggravating your allergies, damaging your immune system, and having other disastrous effects on your health or the health of your family, including children and unborn fetuses.

Many people regularly spray their homes with air fresheners and disinfectant sprays, or light scented candles and fill bowls with potpourri. Although these substances may seem harmless enough, most of them have not undergone a single safety test. Many of the chemicals with which they are made were classified by the US and Canadian governments as "generally recognized as safe" (GRAS), even though they were never subjected to safety testing. Independent organizations and laboratories are revealing that these so-called safe products are not so safe at all. And when you're trying to heal from allergies, it is important to replace toxic chemicals with more natural ones.

The Natural Resources Defense Council (NRDC), an international nonprofit environmental organization, conducted a study of "air fresheners," "air sanitizers," and other related products called "Clearing the Air: Hidden Hazards of Air Fresheners" in which they found that 86 percent of readily available air fresheners tested contained dangerous phthalates.[1] Additionally, none of the products tested listed phthalates on the label, even though they are linked to serious health concerns.

Phthalates are used as plastic softeners; antifoaming agents in aerosols; in vinyl found in children's toys, automobiles, paints, pesticides; and in cosmetics and fragrances. Use of phthalates since World War II has risen dramatically alongside the increased incidence of allergies.

Additionally, the NRDC research found that "most phthalates are well known to interfere with production of the male hormone testosterone, and have been associated with reproductive abnormalities."

Numerous other animal studies have also shown that exposure to phthalates decreases testosterone, causes malformations of the genitalia, and reduced sperm production. Human studies link phthalates to changes in hormones, poor semen quality, and changes in genital formation. Five phthalates, including one found in air fresheners, are listed by the state of California as "known to cause birth defects or reproductive harm." Additionally, phthalates in air fresheners are associated with allergic symptoms and asthma, according to the NRDC.

To test a possible correlation between phthalate exposures and incidence of allergies, researchers at the Swedish National Testing and Research Institute assessed 10,852 children and determined that 198 children had the most persistent allergy symptoms; 202 additional children without allergies acted as controls for the study. Then the researchers assessed the concentration of phthalates found in dust collected from their homes. They found that those children with the worst allergies also had the highest levels of phthalates in their homes, suggesting a link between these toxic chemicals and allergies. They found that butyl benzyl phthalate (BBzP), a type of phthalate, was associated with allergic rhinitis (nasal congestion) and eczema, whereas another type of phthalate known as di(2-ethylhexyl) phthalate (DEHP) was associated with allergy-induced asthma. They published their findings in the medical journal *Environmental Health Perspectives*.[2]

Research by the US Centers for Disease Control and Prevention (CDC) found that the majority of the American population is routinely exposed to at least five different phthalates. Their research also shows that even if the exposures are small—and they may not be!—there is a significant health threat due to the combination of phthalates creating a higher dose.

Hitting the Wal

No, that's not a typo. When I say "hitting the wal" in the context of air fresheners, I'm referring to the extremely high amounts of phthalates the NRDC found in the Walgreens Air Freshener and Walgreens Scented Bouquet along with Ozium Glycol-ized Air Sanitizer. All three of these products had more than 100ppm— considered a high amount for exposure. Walgreens Scented Bouquet Air Freshener had an alarming 7300ppm!

But Walgreens and Ozium aren't the only culprits. Here are the amounts of phthalates found by the NRDC in some of the common air fresheners:[3]

Walgreens Scented Bouquet Air Freshener: 7300ppm of DEP; 0.47ppm of DBP; 6.5ppm DMP
Walgreens Air Freshener Spray: 1100ppm of DEP
Ozium Glycol-ized Air Sanitizer: 360ppm DEP; 0.15ppm DMP
Glade PlugIns Scented Oil: 4.5ppm DBP
Glade Air Infusions: 1.5 ppm DEP
Air Wick Scented Oil: 0.75ppm DBP; 6.3ppm DEP; 1.6ppm DIBP; 2.1ppm DIHP
Febreze NOTICEables Scented Oil: 0.19ppm DBP; 1.5ppm DIBP

Additionally, new scientific research has been disproving the outdated belief that "the dose makes the poison"—in other words, the notion that you have to have a high toxic exposure to have harmful health effects. With the advent of newer testing equipment along with greater volumes of research, scientists have disproved this belief, particularly with hormone disruptors. Sometimes even seemingly miniscule amounts can have serious health consequences.

It's easy to simply stop buying and using "air fresheners," "air sanitizers," and "air deodorizers." Even many "natural" or "unscented products" simply use extra ingredients to mask the scents. So make your home, car, and office off-limits to so-called air fresheners. If you're not the one in charge at your office, show your boss this information and request that they enact such a policy for the sake of everyone in your office or workplace.

If you're trying to improve the smell of your home, car, or workplace, open a window to let some fresh air inside. Put a few drops of natural essential oils—not the same as fragrance oils, which are synthetic toxins—on your damp dust rag, and wipe household and furniture surfaces with it. Alternatively, use an aromatherapy diffuser that sprays natural, essential oils into the air. Better yet, choose from the essential oils outlined in chapter 7 to give your home a pleasing smell and your body a dose of allergy-alleviating essential oils.

The NRDC study also found many toxic ingredients other than phthalates, including acetone, butane (yes, that's lighter fluid!), liquefied petroleum gas, propane, and formaldehyde, among many others, which are all linked to respiratory problems.

> *Acetone* is a respiratory, blood, heart, gastrointestinal, liver, kidney, skin, brain, and nervous system toxin. In other words, it can damage just about any part of your body and have a wide range of adverse effects, including many allergic symptoms.
>
> *Butane* and *Isobutane*. Yes, lighter fluid. It's a serious toxin to the brain and nervous systems. Because the brain plays a significant role in balancing our body chemistry linked to allergies, this toxin is best avoided.

Liquefied Petroleum Gas and Petroleum Distillate. It is fairly obvious why we wouldn't want to add this to our air supply. I've been half-jokingly telling my clients for years that air fresheners contain the by-products of gasoline that the oil industry can't put into vehicles. From the research, it looks like my jokes were not far from the truth.

Propane is a respiratory, skin, cardiovascular and blood, liver, kidney, and nervous system toxin that's known to be extremely dangerous. This is why we operate propane barbecues outdoors, yet we're spraying this stuff into our indoor air.

Perfume. This single ingredient contains up to four hundred different toxic ingredients, 95 percent of which are derived from petroleum products and are linked to a whole list of serious health conditions, ranging from allergies and headaches and dizziness to depression and behavioral changes.

Benzene is known to cause respiratory issues as well as leukemia in humans.

Formaldehyde is linked to respiratory problems and cancers of the upper airways.

So open a window and let in some fresh air rather than resorting to toxic chemical sprays or plug-in products. If outdoor allergens are the issue for you, use the aromatherapy oils I discussed in the last chapter. Unlike the chemical air fresheners, these oils actually freshen and improve air quality while improving your health at the same time.

What About That Car Air Freshener?

Can't smell the forest for the tree air freshener hanging from the rearview mirror? That's the concern of more and more people who report allergies, sinus congestion, headaches, dizziness, and other negative symptoms from the "air fresheners" that hang in vehicles to mask odors.

It has been my concern since I bought a small used pickup truck a few years back. It came complete with manual transmission, CD player, canopy, and the classic cardboard tree hanging from the rearview mirror. Almost immediately I had a severe headache and allergy symptoms from the scent emanating from the truck. I assumed that once I chopped that tree from the windshield the truck would lose its awful scent and the headache and allergy symptoms would be gone. A year later, after cleaning the upholstery with a homemade, all-natural brew and keeping the windows down every day to air it out, I still couldn't drive that truck without feeling nauseated and headachy. Now, I'm not suggesting it was due to a single scented cardboard tree, as I'm sure it had been sprayed with other "air fresheners" and car-detailing products, but it raises the question: *Just what is in that tree?*

A consumer relations specialist at Car-Freshner Corporation (that's no typo—that's actually the spelling) in Watertown, New York—the official manufacturer of scented trees products for cars—said in a recent newspaper article, "I can't tell you what's in them because it's proprietary information."[4] This is a legal loophole that many companies exploit in the name of "trade secrets." Although a combination of ingredients is actually a patent or trade secret, not a trademark, I have no doubt that the company is vigilant about protecting the blend of ingredients it uses in its products. After all, it has been in business for more than sixty years, and consumers still have no idea what they are breathing when they hang a tree in their vehicle.

According to the corporate website, the American company founder Julius Sämann had lived in the Canadian pine forests extracting aromatic oils before inventing the hanging "air freshener." Having lived in pine forests all over Canada, I can say with some degree of confidence that I've never smelled one that made me nauseated, gave me headaches, made me dizzy, or made it hard for me to breathe. Actually, my regular walks in the Canadian pine forests have always eliminated headaches, helped me feel clearer, and helped deepen my breathing.

I can't speak to what Car-Freshner's little trees contain, and maybe we'll never know, thanks to regulators that allow trade secrets to take priority over public health and consumers' right to know what they are buying and breathing. I can, however, tell you that like some of the research I shared above about the number and severity of toxic ingredients in common air fresheners, it is highly likely that some or all of these chemicals are used in car plug-ins and other car air-freshening products. Don't be duped by the advertising slogans like Febreze's that say, "Go on, breathe happy." You won't breathe happy with the use of these products. You'll be far more likely to suffer from the sinus congestion, asthma, and other respiratory problems linked to the toxic chemicals found in many of these products.

WHAT'S LURKING IN FEBREZE?

Forget what the TV commercials tell you: Febreze doesn't contain some miracle substance that envelopes bacteria midair, leaving your house sanitized, fresh, and clean smelling. And it doesn't help you overcome some ridiculous made-up health condition the manufacturers call "noseblindness." What it really does may disturb you, however. Proctor and Gamble discloses only three ingredients on their Febreze-brand products, yet the Environmental Working Group (EWG), an American-based nonprofit that advocates for health protection, found a whopping eighty-nine chemicals in Febreze Air Effects.[5] According to the EWG study, the following are some of the toxic chemicals found in this Febreze product:

BHT is a known neurotoxin (a substance that is toxic to the brain and nervous system), a hormone disruptor, immune system toxin, and irritant to the skin, eyes, and lungs.

Acetaldehyde is a known carcinogen—it causes cancer—that has reproductive and development effects (yes, that means it can damage a fetus) and is an immune system toxin and irritant to the skin, eyes, and lungs.

Fragrance is one of the three disclosed ingredients. However, on its own, it can contain up to four hundred ingredients, most of which are petrochemicals. Clinical observation by medical doctors has found that exposure to fragrances can damage the central nervous system and cause depression, hyperactivity, irritability, inability to cope, behavioral damages, headaches, dizziness, rashes, hyperpigmentation, vomiting, coughing, and skin irritation. A shocking 95 percent of the chemicals used as "fragrance" are derived from petroleum. According to the research of Julia Kendall (available at www.ehnca.org), the most common chemicals in fragrances are ethanol, benzaldehyde, benzyl acetate, a-pinene, acetone, benzyl alcohol, ethyl acetate, linalool, a-terpinene, methylene chloride, and a-terpineol.

Propylene Glycol, also a known carcinogen, is toxic to the immune system and linked to allergies, and it accumulates in the body and irritates the eyes, lungs, and skin.

1,3-Dichloro-2-propanol causes cancer.

Limonene is an allergen, immune system toxin, and skin, lungs, and eye irritant.

Methyl Pyrrolidone is a reproductive system toxin linked to birth defects, allergies, immune system toxicity, and skin, eyes, and lung irritation.

Alcohol, Denatured, is also one of the three disclosed ingredients in Febreze. In this form, it is linked to cancer, birth defects, organ system toxicity, and skin, eye, and lung irritation.

Butylphenyl Methylpropional is an allergen, irritant, and immune system toxin.

Ethyl Acetate, another neurotoxin, is also linked to developmental and reproductive toxicity.

Benzaldehyde is also a neurotoxin and skin, lung, and eye irritator.

Of course, the list goes on and on. The previous slogan for Febreze is "We're out to make the world breathe happy," and now it is "Go on, breathe happy." When I read the ingredient list and their toxic effects, I'm not breathing happy, and I doubt you are either.

Obviously, the biggest issue is that these ingredients really shouldn't be allowed in products that will be sprayed into the air, inhaled, or absorbed directly into the bloodstream through skin contact. But there are other issues, like duping the public into thinking that these products are somehow cleaning the air and eliminating odors. They simply mask them.

As for the toxic effects, Proctor and Gamble also offers a wide selection of drugs that can address many of the symptoms and conditions linked to Febreze ingredients. Can you say "conflict of interest" faster than you can send a toxic whiff of Febreze into the air?

As if spraying this stuff around the house wasn't enough, now household garbage just got a lot more disgusting. The Glad Products Company, the makers of Glad garbage bags, decided it wasn't enough that people are breathing Febreze in so-called air fresheners, so they've started adding it to their garbage bags as well under the guise of "OdorShield."

The Glad Products Company states on its website, "Glad is committed to doing everything we can to create a better environment for generations to come." You might disagree now that you know about the chemicals in their Febreze-infused garbage bags. So while you're avoiding chemical air fresheners, it is also important to avoid the same chemicals in garbage bags. Choose brands that do not use chemical air fresheners or scents.

One study found that being exposed to so-called air fresheners as little as once a week can increase your odds of developing asthma by as much as 71 percent and can contribute to an increase in pulmonary diseases.[6] The same study found that people with high blood levels of the chemical 1,4-dichlorobenzene, which is commonly found in air fresheners, were more likely to experience a decline in lung function.

Many air fresheners and metered disinfectant pumps come with warning labels that state "Deliberately . . . inhaling the vapor of the contents may be harmful or fatal" or "Avoid inhaling spray mist or vapor."

We've been duped into thinking that we need these products to protect us from harmful bacteria or viruses, even though there is no evidence that they actually disinfect the air at all. However, the evidence is mounting that these chemical products harm us . . . sometimes irreparably.

Before you assume that the natural options aren't as effective, think again. This is a marketing myth perpetuated by the companies who manufacture these products, and it couldn't be further from the truth. Many natural options are significantly superior to the toxic chemical options. I've shared some recipes for healthier allergy-reducing cleaning and air-freshening products in chapter 9, Recipes for Allergy Relief.

CLEANING HOUSE

There are many harmful ingredients found in commonly available cleaning products, ingredients that can cause or aggravate many allergy symptoms. As a result, they are best avoided, as they can overburden the immune and respiratory systems that are already overwhelmed during allergy season. Many of the products we rely on simply aren't safe enough for our use.

The EWG commissioned a study of the twenty-one most commonly used cleaning products used in California schools—and it is highly likely that these are the same products used elsewhere in America and around the world. They used a leading laboratory specializing in air pollution released by cleaning products. What they found may alarm you.

- Comet Disinfectant Powder Cleanser emitted the most chemicals, at 146 contaminants released. The fewest contaminants detected were found in Glance NA, a certified green glass and general purpose cleaner, which emitted only one contaminant.

- Twenty-four of the chemicals in the cleaning products have well-established links to asthma, cancer, and other serious health concerns.
- Twelve of the chemicals are on the state of California's Proposition 65, chemicals that are linked to birth defects, reproductive toxicity, and cancer.
- Ten products—Alpha HP, Citrus-Scrub, Comet, Febreze Air Effects, Goof Off, Pine-Sol, Pioneer Super Cleaner, Shineline Seal, Simple Green, and Waxie Green— contained at least one of the developmentally damaging and cancer- or birth defect–causing chemicals on the Californian list.
- Cleaning products that weren't certified green released an average of thirty-eight different contaminants each— almost five times higher than certified green ones that released an average of eight contaminants each.
- Certified green cleaning products contained one-quarter of the chemicals linked to asthma and cancer than the noncertified cleaning products.
- The laboratory determined that cleaning classrooms with certified green products releases less than one-sixth of the air pollution as conventional cleaners.

To help you detox your home and the air you breathe, I've compiled the most common cleaning products, the worst offending chemicals typically found in each, the best all-natural ingredients that you can use in place of the chemicals, and, in chapter 9, a recipe for each cleaning product so you can make your home as healthy as possible.

ALL-PURPOSE CLEANERS

Uses: All-purpose cleaning products are typically used to clean countertops, sinks, tiles, tubs, and floors. Although it tends to be used for many different purposes, hence the name, it isn't suitable for floors, windows, glass, or mirrors.

Worst Ingredient: **Butyl cellosolve**, which is common in all-purpose, window, and other types of cleaners. It can damage bone marrow, the nervous system, kidneys, and the liver.[7]

Better Ingredient Choices: Castile soap and hot water.

Castile soap is named after an olive-growing region in Spain. It was typically made with olive oil and animal fat, but many newer and superior varieties contain plant-based palm, coconut, hemp, or jojoba. Not all castile soap is created equally, so be sure to choose a product that is free from processed detergents and animal products. Check out the recipe for an All-Natural All-Purpose Cleaner on page 182.

ALL-PURPOSE SCRUB

Uses: Powdered all-purpose scrubs are typically used for cleaning sinks, tiles, and bathtubs.

Worst Ingredient: **Chlorinated phenols** found in toilet bowl cleaners are toxic to the respiratory and circulatory systems.[8]

Better Ingredient Choice: Baking soda.

Baking soda is a type of salt known as sodium bicarbonate. On its own, it can lift dirt and deodorize and whiten fabrics or household surfaces, making it a great choice for an all-purpose cleaner. It has a gritty texture, which makes it perfect when you need a scouring scrub.

GLASS AND WINDOW CLEANER

Uses: Windows, mirrors, and car windshields.
Worst Ingredient: **Diethylene glycol** found in window cleaners depresses the nervous system.
Better Ingredient Choice: White vinegar.

White vinegar, which is also known as acetic acid, is a natural disinfectant, deodorizer, and grease cutter. According to the well-known environmental group the David Suzuki Foundation, it kills *E. coli*, salmonella, and other bacteria, making it a great all-natural disinfectant.[9]

LAUNDRY SOAP

Uses: Cleaning clothes, bedding, bath towels, and cloths.
Worst Ingredient: **Nonylphenol ethoxylate**, a common surfactant (detergent) found in laundry detergents and all-purpose cleaners, is banned in Europe; it has been shown to biodegrade slowly into even more toxic compounds.[10]
Better Ingredient Choice: Washing soda.

Washing soda is a type of salt known as sodium carbonate and is a relative of baking soda except that it is more alkaline than its cousin. Although it is natural, even some natural substances can be damaging if ingested, so it should be kept away from children and pets. Clearly label all products made with washing soda.

STAIN REMOVER

Uses: Pretreating fabrics and clothing to remove difficult stains.
Worst Ingredient: **Perchloroethylene**, a chemical spot remover,
   causes liver and kidney damage.[11]
Better Ingredient Choice: Orange oil.

Orange oil is extracted from the skins of oranges, and just a few drops work well as a stain remover when pretreating clothes or other fabrics. Do a test patch on a hidden part of the clothing or fabric to ensure the orange oil won't remove the fabric dye. Orange oil is available in most health food stores. Keep it and products made with it away from children and pets, and label products accordingly. Do not ingest.

ROOM DISINFECTANT

Uses: Deodorizing and disinfecting household air.
Worst Ingredients: **Formaldehyde**, found in spray and wick
   deodorizers, is a respiratory irritant and suspected carcinogen,[12] and benzene in air "fresheners" has been linked
   to leukemia. **Phenols** found in disinfectants are toxic to
   respiratory and circulatory systems.[13] Butane—yes, lighter
   fluid—is found in many air fresheners and disinfecting
   sprays and is a respiratory, brain, and nervous system toxin.
Better Ingredient Choices: Essential oils of thyme, oregano,
   and tea tree.

Thyme and oregano show significant antimicrobial activity against pneumonia, strep, and staphylococcus bacteria, among others.[14] Tea tree oil has strong antibacterial, antiviral, and anti-fungal properties.[15]

THE DIRTY DOZEN CLEANING PRODUCTS

It's easy to overlook cleaning products as the culprit behind health problems. After all, they're improving the cleanliness of our homes, aren't they? According to the EWG, they are frequently causing more harm than good, including many respiratory and skin symptoms that mimic allergies and may potentially aggravate allergic symptoms, among other health issues. The organization routinely examines cleaning products to determine the worst health offenders. Although this is not an exhaustive list, here are some of the worst culprits that made EWG's Cleaners Database Hall of Shame (in alphabetical order, not order of toxicity):[16]

Air Wick. Also designed for spraying into the air we breathe, this "air freshener" carries the warning about the dangers of inhaling the product being harmful or fatal.

CVS/pharmacy Fume-Free Oven Cleaner. Although the product's name suggests it is free of toxic fumes, the label warns "vapor harmful . . . open windows and doors or use other means to ensure fresh air entry during application and drying." The label also indicates that the product contains a substance "known to the state of California to cause cancer." That doesn't exactly sound fume-free, does it?

DampRid Mildew Stain Remover Plus Blocker. This cleaning product may contain up to 10 percent of 2-butoxyethanol, which is a solvent known to be hazardous to health and banned in cleaning products sold in the European Union (EU).

Drano Professional Strength Kitchen Crystals Clog Remover. The product can severely burn eyes and skin and can cause blindness or death. According to the EWG, the product can remain in the drain after use, creating the potential for "extreme hazard."

EASY-OFF Fume Free Oven Cleaner. Like Mop & Glo and Scrubbing Bubbles, this product contains between 5 and 10 percent of butoxydiglycol (sometimes called DEGME), much higher than the 3 percent maximum amount allowed in the EU due to its ability to harm the lungs.

Glade. Although the product is designed to be sprayed into the air we inhale, the warning on the label says it all: "Intentional misuse by deliberately concentrating and inhaling the contents can be harmful or fatal."

Mop & Glo Multi-Surface Floor Cleaner. Mop & Glo also contains DEGME at concentrations up to fifteen times the allowable amount in the European Union. The United Nations Economic Commission for Europe indicates that this chemical is "suspected of damaging the unborn child."

Old English Furniture Polish. Like Glade and Air Wick, this product carries the same warning about being harmful or fatal.

Scrubbing Bubbles. Although the manufacturer's ad may show cute-looking cartoon bubbles working hard to clean bathrooms, this product contains up to 10 percent of DEGME, a solvent that is banned in concentrations over 3 percent in the EU. It causes lung irritation and inflammation.

Spic and Span Multi-Surface and Floor Cleaner. This cleaning product contains nonylphenol ethoxylate, which is banned in the EU and cannot be used in cleaning products manufactured after 2012 in California. It can disrupt hormones and is toxic to aquatic life and is persistent in the environment.

Spot Shot. Spot Shot also advises that "inhalation abuse of aerosol products may be harmful or fatal," although the product is designed for spraying into the air we breathe.

Walmart Great Value Heavy Duty Oven Cleaner. Your body may not find this product to be such a great value. The label indicates that it "will burn skin and eyes. Avoid contact with skin, eyes, mucous membranes and clothing. Harmful if swallowed. Avoid inhaling spray mist." Anyone who has ever used a chemical oven cleaner knows that it is hard to avoid inhaling it, particularly when it is sitting in your oven. And there is obviously a reason to avoid inhaling it, or else the company would not add this disclaimer to their packaging.

CHOOSING BETTER PERSONAL-CARE PRODUCTS

Air fresheners and cleaning products aren't the only products initiating or aggravating allergy symptoms or causing the immune and respiratory systems to malfunction. Personal-care products such as perfumes, hair care, cosmetics, and other products can be a problem as well.

Perfume Pollution

If you've walked through a department store lately, you may have been overwhelmed by the perfume section. Whether you are obsessed with Obsession, a believer in Believe, or consumed by L'Air du Temps, the smell of perfumes and colognes can be overwhelming. The toxic effects of fragrances can be overwhelming as well.

There are more than four hundred potential chemicals that can be used under the single name "fragrance" found on the label of many products, not just perfumes and colognes. Fragrances are found in "air fresheners," room deodorizers, cosmetics, fabric softeners, laundry detergents, candles, and many other products. Manufacturers are not required to list ingredients on the labels of these products, nor do they have to reveal the specific ingredients that qualify as "fragrance" to regulating authorities because they are protected as trade secrets.

Some of the most common chemicals in perfumes are ethanol, acetaldehyde, benzaldehyde, benzyl acetate, a-pinene, acetone, benzyl alcohol, ethyl acetate, linalool, a-terpinene, methylene chloride, styrene oxide, dimethyl sulphate, a-terpineol, camphor, and limonene. Some of these chemicals cause asthma, burning or itching skin irritations, coughing, eye irritation, fatigue, headaches, and sinus pain, all of which may seem similar to allergic reactions. Some of the other problems linked to these chemicals include irritability, mental vagueness, muscle pain, bloating, joint aches, sore throat, gastrointestinal problems, laryngitis, dizziness, swollen lymph nodes, and spikes in blood pressure.

And that's just the tip of the iceberg. Acetaldehyde is a probable human carcinogen. In animal studies, it crosses the placenta to a fetus. The chemical industry's own Toxic Data Safety Sheets list headaches, tremors, convulsions, and even death as a possible effect of exposure to acetonitrile, another common fragrance ingredient. In animal studies, styrene oxide causes depression. Toluene, also known as methyl benzene, is a well-established neurotoxin that can cause loss of muscle control, brain damage, headaches, memory loss, and problems with speech, hearing, and vision. Musk tetralin has been shown to cause brain cell and spinal cord degeneration.

Research confirms that many of the ingredients in fragrances are neurotoxins, meaning that they have poisonous effects on the brain and nervous system. Additional studies link other negative emotional, mental, and physical symptoms to various fragrance ingredients. Until recently, scientists believed that the brain was protected by an impermeable mechanism known as the *blood-brain barrier*. This is only partly true. Recent studies show that this system allows many environmental toxins, including those found in perfumes and other scented products, access to the delicate brain and that once found in the brain, it can take decades to eliminate—decades that can result in substantial damage in the form of inflammation and plaque build-up in the brain, two of the precursors to serious brain disorders like Alzheimer's and Parkinson's.

Some fragrance ingredients disrupt our natural hormonal balance, causing any number of possible emotional concerns, including anxiety, mood swings, and depression. Feeling down? It could be the scent you're wearing. Even if you can't pick up the scent of perfumes, you may be suffering ill effects from exposure.

Not all scented products were created equally. Commercial brands of perfumes and colognes are primarily composed of

synthetic chemicals. Even many natural products contain synthetic fragrance ingredients, so it's important to start reading
labels on personal-care products. If there is no ingredient list,
the manufacturer may have something to hide. Also, beware of
fragrance oils masquerading as essential oils. The former is synthetic, whereas the latter are derived from flowers, leaves, and
other natural substances.

Shakespeare claimed, "That which we call a rose by any other
name would smell as sweet." Thanks to today's chemical industry, that is no longer true. Worse than that, the potential health
effects are anything but sweet. Choose a blend of all-natural
essential oils instead of perfumes, colognes, and other scented
products. Your body will thank you for making the switch.

THE SHOCKING TRUTH ABOUT DIESEL EMISSIONS

You may recall the recent news stories about the automaker Volkswagen (VW) that intentionally violated emissions standards,
according to new information released by the US Environmental
Protection Agency (EPA). On the heels of that announcement,
numerous other vehicle manufacturers were found to be following the same illegal and unethical practice. Although the focus
of the news stories was about the investigations and potential
lawsuits, there is a serious threat that was largely overlooked by
the media: nitrogen oxide pollution from vehicle emissions has
been linked to asthma and other respiratory diseases.

The EPA has ordered VW to fix almost five hundred thousand
cars after discovering that the automaker intentionally misled
regulators by using software that evades EPA standards. The company also faces the potential for $15 billion in fines, although the
exact amount has not yet been announced.[17] Additionally, the US
Justice Department has launched a criminal probe into the rigged
emissions tests, and several law firms have announced plans for

class-action lawsuits against the Volkswagen Group of America. While investigations and lawsuits against the company are under way, the company could still be given up to a year to formulate a plan to correct the substandard vehicles.

In the meantime, numerous vehicle manufacturers have been selling vehicles that exceeded the EPA standards by up to forty times the maximum allowable emissions for nitrogen oxide. According to the Union of Concerned Scientists, a group of scientists and engineers who conduct independent research and attempt to solve the problems facing the planet (including air pollution), diesel emissions account for two-thirds of particulate matter in the air.[18] Particulate from diesel contains hundreds of chemical elements, including sulfate, ammonium, carcinogens, and heavy metals like cadmium and arsenic. There are different sizes of particulate matter, including coarse particulate (less than 10 microns in diameter), fine particulate (less than 2.5 microns), and ultrafine particulate (less than 0.1 microns). Another issue with diesel exhaust is that it is made up of 80 to 95 percent of ultrafine particulate, which is small enough to penetrate lung cells.[19] Everyone is susceptible to diesel soot pollution, but especially those with respiratory concerns like asthma as well as children and the elderly.

Although it is impossible to avoid diesel exhaust or other types of air pollution, if you are suffering from allergies or asthma, it is a good idea to make as much effort as possible to reduce your exposure. Simply turning your car's heat or air conditioning off or setting it to circulate inside your vehicle can reduce your daily exposure. If you own a diesel vehicle, avoid idling it in underground parking areas or in your garage. Better yet, try not to idle it at all. If you are in the market for a new vehicle, an electric, hybrid, or gasoline option is superior to diesel. Additionally, if you are choosing a new place to live, try to avoid areas with high traffic levels, major freeways, industrial parks, or trucking routes if you suffer from allergies or asthma.

NATURAL THERAPIES

We've discussed many highly effective natural therapies to help with allergy and asthma symptoms. But there are some other excellent ones to consider, including nasal rinses and deep breathing exercises.

Rinse Your Nasal Passages

Rinsing your nasal passages with a saltwater solution can help eliminate nasal and sinus congestion while removing any pollens, molds, or other allergens that may be aggravating them. There are multiple ways to rinse out your nasal passageways, including many store-bought, premade nasal sprays. If you choose one of these types of products, be sure to avoid any that contain preservatives or other synthetic chemicals. Most contain salt water only, but there are also some good ones that contain either eucalyptus oil, a natural expectorant that helps clear excess mucus from the sinuses and nasal passageways, or capsaicin, which is the active ingredient in chilies and is highly effective at reducing inflammation in the nasal passageways and sinuses. You can choose one or the other or alternate between them, as their strengths are complementary. If you choose the capsaicin varieties, keep in mind that there is a burning sensation that lasts for about twenty to thirty seconds. I've personally found them intense at first but highly effective. Research has shown that the capsaicin nasal sprays offer dramatic improvement for allergy and rhinitis sufferers.[20]

You can also use a neti pot, which is a small ceramic dish shaped a bit like a gravy boat, to flush your sinuses with a salt-water solution. Most health food stores sell neti pots and saline packets ready to mix with water. You can either follow the package directions or purchase sea salt and mix it with pure warm water. Start with one-quarter teaspoon of sea salt to one cup of water, preferably unchlorinated or filtered water. Simply lean over a sink and tilt your head to the side to pour the water into one nostril and allow it to run out the other nostril. It may take some practice, but it is an excellent way to cleanse and eliminate mucous and microbes. Over time, you can increase to one-half a teaspoon of sea salt per cup of water and cool down the temperature of water you use.

Don't Forget to Breathe

Okay, I know this one sounds obvious, but you'd be surprised how few people actually breathe deeply. And it may seem like an odd thing to mention to people who may be suffering from nasal congestion that makes it difficult to breathe, but it is important to take time out of your day to relax and practice deep breathing. Ideally, use eucalyptus essential oil in a nebulizer or just under your nose in conjunction with your deep breathing exercises. That will help alleviate any nasal congestion that may make it difficult to breathe. You can also rinse your nasal passageways just prior to conducting deep breathing exercises to help make it easier. Don't force your breathing—just follow your natural breathing with a modest effort to deepen it slightly. Deep breathing for even a minute at a time can retrain your body to breathe deeper overall, but it also quickly reduces stress hormones like cortisol that can cause health problems.

TEN HOUSEPLANTS THAT CLEAN THE AIR

Indoor air quality has become a real problem. It often contains formaldehyde from carpets and adhesives, volatile organic compounds from paints, petrochemicals from fragrances, and a laundry list of chemicals from fabric softeners. Although it's always important to let some fresh air in, research by NASA found that many houseplants are capable of reducing harmful toxins in the air, such as benzene, formaldehyde, trichloroethylene (TCE), toluene, and more.

Benzene is a cancer-causing agent found in many glues, solvents, paints, and art supplies. Formaldehyde is a cancer-causing agent that off-gases from furniture and carpets. Trichloroethylene is a solvent used with metal parts, dry cleaning, paints, and paint removers. And toluene is found in nail polish and nail polish remover as well as foam.

Here are ten of the best air-purifying houseplants and the toxins they are most effective at reducing:

1. *Bamboo Palm* (*Chamaedorea seifritzii*): benzene, formaldehyde, TCE

2. *Chrysanthemums or Mums* (*Chrysanthemum morifolium*): benzene, formaldehyde, TCE (most effective against TCE according to NASA)

3. *Common Ivy or English Ivy* (*Hedera helix*): benzene, formaldehyde, TCE, toluene, octane, terpene (most effective against benzene according to NASA)

4. *Ficus Tree or Weeping Fig* (*Ficus benjamina*): benzene, formaldehyde, TCE, octane, terpene

5. *Mass Cane* (*Dracaena massangeana*): benzene, formaldehyde, TCE (most effective against formaldehyde, according to NASA)

6. *Peace Lily* (*Spathiphyllum*): benzene, formaldehyde, TCE

7. *Purple Heart* (*Tradescantia pallida*): benzene, TCE, toluene, terpene

8. *Red Ivy* (*Hemigraphis alternate*): benzene, TCE, toluene, octane, terpene

9. *Spider Plant* (*Chlorophytum comosum, Chlorophytum elatum*): formaldehyde, carbon dioxide, carbon monoxide

10. *Wax Plant* (*Hoya carnosa*): benzene, TCE, toluene, octane, terpene

Of course, if you're prone to dust or mold allergies, you may want to forego the indoor plants. Or if you have allergies to specific indoor plants, I probably don't need to tell you to avoid them.

9

Recipes for Allergy Relief

JUST BECAUSE YOU'LL BE eating an anti-inflammatory diet devoid of dairy and food additives and low in sugar and meat doesn't mean you won't enjoy the many delicious plant-based foods that are part of the *Allergy-Proof Your Life* program. You'll enjoy thirst-quenching juices, savory soups and stews, delicious main dishes, and even decadent desserts as a treat on occasion. Many of my clients are surprised to learn how good these foods can taste. Once you've tried several of the recipes, you'll probably have a good idea of how to apply some of the same principles to your own recipes. Don't be afraid to try new foods, as you may discover some favorites among them.

JUICE, SMOOTHIES, AND TEAS

Carrot-Ginger Anti-inflammatory Juice

Serves 1 to 2

Ginger is a proven anti-inflammatory that helps take down swelling and alleviate sinus pain. Carrots are an excellent source of beta carotene that is needed for a healthy immune system and mucous membranes. Combined they make an excellent juice to help keep allergy symptoms at bay.

  6 large carrots, tops removed
  1 apple, cut into large chunks
  1-inch piece ginger

Pass all ingredients through a juicer. Drink immediately.

Citrus Sensation

Serves 2

The Citrus Sensation gives your body a serious vitamin C boost, which is essential to help heal overtaxed adrenal glands, usually an underlying factor in allergies.

  2 oranges, peeled and sectioned
  2 grapefruit, peeled and sectioned
  ½ lemon, peeled and sectioned
  1 cup water

Juice all citrus ingredients in a citrus or standard juicer. Add water and drink immediately.

Antihistamine Juice

Serves 1 to 2

The beets in this juice contain potent compounds known as anthocyanins, which give foods not only their purplish-red color but also natural anti-inflammatory properties that help reduce the nasal, sinus, and other inflammation linked to allergic reactions.

3 carrots
½ cucumber
½ beet with greens

Juice all ingredients in a juicer. Drink immediately.

Enzyme Power-Healing Smoothie

Serves 1 to 2

Not only is this smoothie delicious and satisfying; it is an amazing healer. Papaya and pineapple are loaded with enzymes that help digestion and break down toxins, fat, and inflammation in the body. Bromelain in pineapple is an excellent all-natural anti-inflammatory that helps heal the gut, a precursor to many allergy symptoms. Papain, an enzyme that is plentiful in papaya, breaks down protein molecules in the blood, including inflammation that is linked to allergies. Enjoy this smoothie as an occasional treat rather than a daily beverage since the pineapple and papaya have a lot of natural sugars that when drunk regularly can have the reverse effect.

1 cup chopped papaya
1 cup chopped fresh pineapple (not canned)
4 ice cubes
water as needed

Blend the papaya, pineapple, and ice cubes. Add water for desired smoothie consistency.

The Decongester

Serves 1

I call this juice The Decongester because both pineapple and ginger help alleviate inflammation and promote gut health, while the ginger adds some spice that helps clear sinuses.

½ pineapple, outer skin removed (juice the core as well as
    the flesh)
1-inch piece ginger
water as needed

Pass all ingredients through a juicer. Dilute with pure water to taste. Drink immediately.

Lemonade Delight

Serves 4

Most bottled lemonade is full of sugar, the consumption of which is a factor for allergies. But you won't miss it once you taste this delicious and superhealthy version. Unlike most sweetened lemonade, thanks to the naturally sweet herb stevia, this lemonade keeps blood sugar levels stable. It tastes so good, even kids will love it.

5 lemons
1½ teaspoons liquid stevia (approximately 90 drops),
    or more for a sweeter lemonade
6 cups pure water
ice cubes for serving
fresh mint, optional, as garnish

Juice the lemons using a wooden or ceramic lemon juicer or an electric citrus juicer if you have one. Pour the juice into a large pitcher.

Add the stevia and top with water. Stir to mix.

Pour over ice and add mint leaves, if using, to garnish. Serve.

GI Soothing Tea

Makes ¾ cup

All three of the ingredients in this warming tea work to soothe the gastrointestinal tract—the source of most inflammation in the body—while the peppermint also helps decongest the sinuses. These dried herbs can be found in most health food stores.

¼ cup dried peppermint
¼ cup dried ginger
¼ cup dried globe artichoke
stevia as needed

Mix the dried herbs in a jar.

Add one teaspoon of the mixture per cup of tea to a tea strainer or tea ball. Pour boiling water over the tea strainer and let sit for five minutes. Sweeten with 1 to 3 drops of stevia per cup if desired.

Almond Cream

Makes approximately 1 cup

Instead of milk, cream, or creamers for your coffee or over oatmeal, cereal, or fruit, try this simple and delicious almond cream.

23 raw almonds
½ cup water
½ teaspoon maple syrup

Place all ingredients in a blender and blend until smooth.

SALADS, SALAD DRESSINGS, AND DIPS

Blueberry Anti-inflammatory Salad Dressing

Makes approximately 1½ cups

Both blueberries and flaxseed oil are excellent anti-inflammatory agents. Blueberries contain a substance that is ten times more potent than aspirin at fighting pain and inflammation.

When choosing apple cider vinegar, be sure to choose a brand that has sediment at the bottom, most easily found at a health food store. And double-check that your maple syrup is the real deal, not maple flavored or other types of syrup products, most of which do not contain actual maple syrup.

    ½ cup blueberries, fresh or frozen
    ¾ cup cold-pressed flaxseed oil (make sure it is
        refrigerated)
    ⅓ cup apple cider vinegar
    dash Celtic sea salt
    1 teaspoon pure maple syrup

Blend with a hand mixer or whisk together. If whisking ingredients together, mash the blueberries with a fork. Pour over mixed baby greens or your preferred type of salad greens.

Herb Salad Dressing

Makes approximately 1 cup

Forget store-bought salad dressings. This one is a cinch and takes only a couple of minutes to whip up. Its fresh and savory flavor makes a great addition to any salad. It also works well on chopped salads—the kind with lots of chopped vegetables—or quinoa salads with fresh veggies.

When choosing apple cider vinegar, be sure to choose a brand that has sediment at the bottom, most easily found at a health food store.

¾ cup cold-pressed flaxseed oil (make sure it is
    refrigerated)
⅓ cup apple cider vinegar
½ teaspoon Celtic sea salt
½ teaspoon basil
½ teaspoon thyme
½ teaspoon oregano
dash cayenne pepper

Whisk all ingredients together or place in a jar and shake together. Pour over fresh mesclun salad greens (mixed baby greens) and enjoy!

Sweet Greens Wild Berry Dressing

Makes approximately 1 cup

My sister, the owner of Sweet Greens Juice Bar and Café in Hagersville, Ontario, Canada, shared her delicious salad dressing recipe.

½ cup mixed berries, fresh or frozen
1 tablespoon honey
1 tablespoon extra-virgin olive oil
3 tablespoons fresh lemon juice
1 tablespoon orange juice

Blend and pour on your favorite salad greens.

Mom's Amazing Coleslaw

Serves 4

This delicious coleslaw is devoid of the typical inflammation-causing mayonnaise dressings in favor of a lighter, anti-inflammatory one. The apples and raisins add some natural sweetness without excessively loading it with sugar like most coleslaw does. But the healthy spin on this salad doesn't affect how great it tastes.

When choosing apple cider vinegar, be sure to choose a brand that has sediment at the bottom, most easily found at a health food store.

COLESLAW

½ cabbage, grated
2 carrots, grated
¼ onion, finely grated or chopped
1 celery stalk, finely chopped
¼ cup organic raisins
1 apple, grated, optional

DRESSING

½ cup extra-virgin olive oil
3 tablespoons unpasteurized honey
¼ cup apple cider vinegar

Mix all coleslaw ingredients together in a bowl.

Mix together dressing ingredients in a jar and shake until blended.

Pour dressing over coleslaw until well mixed. Serve.

Protein-Packed Bean Salad

Serves 4

This salad is high in protein and fiber, as I'm sure you will discover within a day or so of eating it. It is anti-inflammatory and helps restore gut health, but you'll also enjoy its delicious taste.

When choosing apple cider vinegar, be sure to choose a brand that has sediment at the bottom, most easily found at a health food store. And double-check that your maple syrup is the real deal, not maple flavored or other types of syrup products, most of which do not contain actual maple syrup.

> one 14-ounce can cooked mixed beans (e.g., kidney, garbanzo, pinto, etc.), rinsed and drained
> 2 celery stalks, finely chopped
> ¼ purple onion, finely chopped
> ½ green bell pepper, finely chopped
> ½ red bell pepper, finely chopped
> 1 green onion, finely chopped
> ¾ cup cold-pressed flaxseed oil (make sure it is refrigerated)
> ⅓ cup apple cider vinegar
> ½ teaspoon Celtic sea salt
> 1 tablespoon pure maple syrup
> ½ teaspoon basil
> ½ teaspoon thyme
> ½ teaspoon oregano
> dash cayenne pepper

Mix the beans and vegetables together in a bowl.

Whisk together in a separate bowl or jar the oil, vinegar, salt, syrup, herbs, and cayenne pepper.

Pour half of the dressing over the bean and vegetable mixture. For best taste, let marinate overnight or a couple of hours.

Store the remaining dressing in a covered jar in the refrigerator for later use.

Guacamole Salad

Serves 2 to 4

This is one of my favorite salads. It is refreshing and delicious and perfect for a hot summer night when the tomatoes are coming out of the garden or farmer's markets. But it is so tasty, you'll want to enjoy it year-round.

> 1 head leaf or romaine lettuce, washed and dried
> 1 tomato, chopped
> 1 avocado, chopped
> dash Celtic sea salt
> handful fresh cilantro
> 1 tablespoon cold-pressed flaxseed oil
> 1 lime
> 1 small garlic clove

Cut or tear lettuce and place in bowls to form a base for the other salad ingredients.

Place tomato, avocado, salt, cilantro, and oil together in a separate bowl. Squeeze the juice of the lime over the other ingredients. Chop or press garlic into the bowl with the other ingredients. Toss ingredients together. Pour tomato mixture over the salad greens and serve.

Sweet Broccoli Salad

Serves 2 to 4

My sister, Bobbi-Jo Meyer, owner of Sweet Greens Juice Bar and Café in Hagersville, Ontario, Canada, developed and shared this recipe. She was looking for a delicious way to get more antioxidant-rich raw broccoli into her diet and succeeded with this recipe.

SALAD

> 1 head broccoli, finely chopped
> 1 carrot, grated

2 apples, cored and chopped
1 cup raisins
¼ cup raw, unsalted sunflower seeds

DRESSING

½ cup extra-virgin oil or Udo's Special Blend oil
1 tablespoon apple cider vinegar
1 tablespoon unpasteurized honey

Soak raisins in water for at least 30 minutes. Drain and discard water.

Mix all salad ingredients, including raisins, together.

Mix dressing ingredients together.

Pour dressing over vegetable mixture. Toss and enjoy.

Brown Rice and Almond Salad

Serves 2 to 4

When you need a hearty salad, this one does the trick. It's both tasty and filling and helps keep you feeling full for hours thanks to its blood sugar–balancing properties.

SALAD

½ cup almonds, chopped and soaked in water overnight
2 cups cooked brown or wild rice
¾ cup chopped celery
¾ cup chopped red bell pepper
1 green onion, chopped
large handful fresh parsley, chopped

DRESSING

¼ cup extra virgin olive oil or Udo's Special Blend oil
1 to 2 tablespoons wheat-free tamari (available at most
    health food stores)
dash Celtic sea salt

Drain almonds and discard water.

Mix all salad ingredients together.

Mix all dressing ingredients together.

Pour dressing over salad. Toss and enjoy.

SOUPS, STEWS, AND MAINS

Indian Lentil Curry

Serves 4

This Indian curry tastes so fabulous that you may forget there is no meat or dairy in it. It's a staple in our household and one of my husband's favorite dishes. The high amount of fiber helps balance blood sugar, plus it cleanses the intestinal tract of harmful microbes. It is also quick and easy to make.

   1 yam, cubed
   1 large onion, chopped
   ½ teaspoon mustard seeds
   4 dried red chilies
   1-inch piece ginger, grated
   2 garlic cloves, chopped
   2 tablespoons extra-virgin olive oil
   3 cups cooked lentils, or two small cans, rinsed
   ½ teaspoon turmeric
   1 teaspoon Celtic sea salt
   ½ cup water
   fresh cilantro, if desired

Boil the yam in a medium to large pot in water until soft. Pour off excess water, leaving enough to mash the yams with a hand blender until smooth.

Cook the onion, mustard seeds, chilies, ginger, and garlic in the olive oil in a frying pan over low heat until the onion is transparent. Add the onion mixture to the mashed yams.

Add the lentils, turmeric, salt, and water. Stir together. Let simmer over low heat until warmed and flavors mingle.

Serve in bowls with fresh cilantro as a garnish.

Roasted Vegetable and Rosemary Soup

Serves 2 to 4

This is my husband's all-time favorite soup. It is anti-inflammatory and packed with veggies, and the actual preparation time is minimal. You can even roast extra vegetables to keep on hand when you want this soup in a hurry.

MARINADE

    3 tablespoons extra-virgin olive oil
    1 sprig fresh rosemary or 2 teaspoons dried
       rosemary
    1 teaspoon dried thyme
    ½ teaspoon Celtic sea salt

SOUP

    1 sweet potato or yam
    1 red bell pepper
    1 green bell pepper
    2 medium potatoes
    1 large onion
    5 garlic cloves
    1 carrot
    hot water or stock as needed

Mix all marinade ingredients together.

Chop all the vegetables except the garlic into 1-inch pieces and place in a large bowl. Toss with the marinade until coated. (You may need to do this in two stages, depending on the size of the bowl you are using.)

Place all the vegetables, including the garlic, on a large baking tray. Bake at 350°F for 1 hour or until vegetables are soft.

Puree in a food processor or blender, adding hot water or stock to thin to desired consistency. Add Celtic sea salt to taste and serve.

Rich and Savory Wild Rice Soup

Serves 4

Don't worry about the lengthy list of ingredients—this recipe is actually quick and easy to make, particularly if you employ the help of a food processor with the slicing blade intact. It is rich and hearty and perfect for a cool autumn or winter's evening.

    4 garlic cloves, chopped
    1 large onion, chopped
    3 tablespoons extra-virgin olive oil
    8 cups water
    ½ cup wild rice
    1 sweet potato, chopped
    2 celery stalks
    2 carrots, chopped
    4 small red-skinned potatoes, sliced
    ½ cup frozen peas
    3 teaspoons cinnamon
    ½ teaspoon allspice
    1 teaspoon molasses
    2 teaspoons Celtic sea salt, or to taste
    ¼ teaspoon garlic powder
    2 teaspoons cumin
    dash cayenne pepper

1 red bell pepper, sliced

½ cup cooked kidney or pinto beans

Sauté the garlic and onion in the oil in a large pot. When they are slightly browned, add the water and all ingredients through cayenne pepper. Bring to a boil. Once the water begins boiling, turn down the heat and let simmer for 45 minutes.

Add the bell pepper and beans and simmer for an additional 15 minutes or longer, until the vegetables are cooked and the rice is soft. Simmer longer, if desired, to allow flavors to mingle. Stir any spices that sit at the top of the pot into the broth before serving.

Chickpea and Butternut Squash Stew

Serves 2 to 4

I could eat this hearty and anti-inflammatory stew every day— it's that good. But it's equally good for you, thanks to the anti-inflammatory ginger, turmeric, and hot peppers along with the microbe-killing garlic that helps destroy harmful pathogens in the intestines.

2 tablespoons extra-virgin olive oil

1 onion, finely chopped

3 garlic cloves, finely chopped

1 teaspoon finely chopped fresh ginger

1 teaspoon ground turmeric

2 teaspoons ground cumin

½ teaspoon dried hot pepper flakes

3 medium tomatoes, diced

One 13-ounce can chickpeas, drained and rinsed

½ cup organic golden raisins (be sure they do not contain sulfites)

1 cup water

½ medium butternut squash, peeled and cubed

1 red bell pepper, cut into 1-inch slices

Heat oil in a large saucepan. Add the onion and sauté until translucent. Add the garlic and spices and cook for one minute. Add remaining ingredients and bring to a boil, then reduce the heat and simmer for 40 minutes with the lid on. Serve on its own or with rice or couscous.

DESSERTS

Raspberry-Blueberry Ice Cream

Serves 2 to 4

This ice cream is so rich, creamy, and delicious that you won't miss the dairy varieties at all. With this recipe you'll quickly discover that eating an allergy-proof diet does not mean depriving yourself. This ice cream contains powerful natural phytochemicals that help diminish inflammation.

> 1 cup frozen raspberries
> 1 cup frozen blueberries
> 2 frozen bananas

Blend all ingredients in a food processor and serve.

Mixed Berry Pie

Serves 6

This delightful pie is quick and easy to make and just needs a little time to set. The berries give it an anti-inflammatory effect on the body, but you'll probably eat it for the taste alone.

Be sure to double-check that your maple syrup is the real deal, not maple flavored or other types of syrup products, most of which do not contain actual maple syrup. Agar flakes are a form of tasteless seaweed that is packed with nutrients and serves as a thickener; it is available in most health food stores.

CRUST

1 cup rolled oats
½ cup almonds
pinch Celtic sea salt
1 teaspoon cinnamon
1 cup oat flour
⅓ cup coconut oil
2 tablespoons pure maple syrup

FILLING

¼ cup agar flakes
2 cups of unsweetened raspberry, strawberry, mixed berry,
    or apple juice
⅓ cup arrowroot
1 tablespoon maple syrup
4 cups fresh or frozen mixed berries of your choice

For the crust, grind oats, almonds, salt, and cinnamon in a food processor; mix with the flour. Add the oil and syrup and mix to form a soft dough. Press into an oiled and floured 10-inch pie plate and flute the edges if desired. Bake at 350°F for 25 minutes or until golden. Allow to cool while preparing filling.

For the filling, mix agar flakes and juice together in a pot and bring to a rolling boil; boil uncovered for 2 to 3 minutes.

Whisk together the arrowroot and syrup in a small bowl. Add to the juice mixture and whisk constantly until thickened.

Mix berries into the mixture and pour immediately into the pie crust. Refrigerate for 1 to 2 hours or until set. Serve and enjoy!

Coconut Nut Balls

Makes approximately 18 to 20 balls

My sister, Bobbi-Jo Meyer, also shared this quick, simple, and delicious recipe.

Be sure to double-check that your maple syrup is the real deal, not maple flavored or other types of syrup products, most of which do not contain actual maple syrup.

    1 cup raw, unsalted almonds or walnuts, ground
    1 cup unsweetened coconut flakes
    1 cup raw almond butter
    2 tablespoons pure maple syrup
    additional ground nuts or coconut for rolling

Mix all ingredients together in a food processor. Form into small balls and roll in ground nuts or coconut. Serve and enjoy!

Berry "Gelatin"

Serves 6

Typically Jell-O is made from gelatin, which is an animal product. But this gelatin recipe is made with mineral-rich agar, a type of seaweed available in most health food stores. So now you can have your minerals and your Jell-O too.

Be sure to double-check that your maple syrup is the real deal, not maple flavored or other types of syrup products, most of which do not contain actual maple syrup.

    2 cups raspberry or apple juice
    ¼ cup agar flakes
    ⅓ cup arrowroot
    1 tablespoon pure maple syrup, if desired
    4 cups fresh or frozen berries

Whisk together in a pot the juice and agar and bring to a boil on high heat, whisking the entire time. When the juice starts boiling, reduce the heat to medium and continue cooking for 2 to 3 minutes to dissolve the agar.

Mix the arrowroot and maple syrup in a separate bowl until well blended. (If you opt not to use the maple syrup, mix the arrowroot with 2 tablespoons of water instead.)

Pour the arrowroot mixture into the pot with the juice and whisk until thick, approximately 1 minute. Remove from heat, add the berries, and pour into individual glass or ceramic serving cups.

Refrigerate for 1 to 2 hours to set.

Almond-Oat Thumbprint Cookies

Makes approximately 24 cookies

These sweet and tasty cookies are perfect when you want an occasional treat to satisfy your sweet tooth. They are full of fiber and are simple to make as well.

Be sure to double-check that your maple syrup is the real deal, not maple flavored or other types of syrup products, most of which do not contain actual maple syrup.

    1 cup almonds
    1 cup rolled oats
    1¼ cups oat, kamut, spelt, or rice flour
    1 teaspoon cinnamon
    ½ cup pure maple syrup
    ½ cup cold-pressed walnut oil
    ½ cup unsweetened raspberry or strawberry jam

Preheat the oven to 350°F.

Grind the almonds and oats to a fine meal in a food processor. Add the flour, cinnamon, syrup, and oil, and mix until well combined.

Form dough into walnut-sized balls and place on an oiled cookie sheet. Press an indentation in the center of each ball with your thumb and fill indentation with jam. Continue until all dough has been used.

Bake for 10 to 15 minutes or until golden.

CLEANING PRODUCTS

There are more reasons than ever to make your own all-natural cleaning products: not only will you avoid the harmful chemicals found in many commercially available products and reduce the harmful sinus and respiratory effects; you'll save money. You'll also probably be surprised to find that many natural options work better than their chemical counterparts!

Natural All-Purpose Cleaner

Makes approximately 1 gallon

If you're looking for an all-natural all-purpose cleaner that disinfects surfaces and kills harmful bacteria, look no further. Not only is this superior to commercial products, but it is also a lot more affordable too.

  1 gallon hot water
  ½ cup liquid castile soap
  10 drops thyme essential oil

Combine all ingredients and pour into a spray bottle. Shake before using.

Natural All-Purpose Scrub

Makes 3 cups

If you need a cleaning product with some scouring ability, then try this all-purpose scrub. It is great on bathtubs, sinks, tile, and other surfaces.

2 cups baking soda

½ cup liquid castile soap

½ cup water

Mix all ingredients together. Pour into a squirt bottle and shake before each use. Rinse well after use.

Natural Glass Cleaner

Makes 2 cups

Forget commercial window cleaners: vinegar and water work much better, as you'll soon discover once you try it. Plus, it is much cheaper than window-cleaning products. Save a spray bottle to spray this cleaner on windows and mirrors.

1 cup white vinegar

1 cup water

Mix together. Pour into a spray bottle. Shake before using.

Natural Laundry Soap

Makes approximately 2 gallons

Most laundry products are full of chemicals that are damaging to the respiratory system and can aggravate sinus, nasal, and lung concerns. Fortunately it is easy to make your own natural laundry soap.

Borax, or sodium borate, is a natural, alkaline mineral salt. Like washing soda, borax is also best kept away from children and pets and should never be ingested. Label products made with these products accordingly.

7 quarts water

1 cup soap granules

½ cup borax

½ cup washing soda (for hard water, double the amount of washing soda)

20 drops lavender or lemon essential oils, optional (choose
essential oils, not "fragrance oils," which are synthetic)

Mix 1 quart of water with the soap granules in a pot until diluted.

Mix remaining 6 quarts of water, borax, and washing soda in a
clean bucket. Add the water–soap granule mixture and stir until
dissolved; add the oils if using. Soap will thicken as it cools.

Pour into a large container or jar to store.

Natural Stain Remover

Makes 1½ cups

No commercial stain-removing products can compete with the
stain-removing action of this natural option. Not only does it work
marvelously, but it smells great too. Be sure to test for colorfast-
ness on a hidden part of your garment before using it on stains.

1 cup water
½ cup orange oil

Mix ingredients together and pour into a spray bottle. Spray
stains with the solution prior to adding to the washing machine.

Natural Room Disinfectant

Makes approximately 2 cups

Forget the chemical-laden air "fresheners" or deodorizers available on the market—this one contains three different proven
disinfecting essential oils that work as well or better than the
chemical options but don't cause the respiratory damage that
the chemical varieties do.

2 cups water
15 drops thyme essential oil
15 drops tea tree essential oil

10 drops oregano essential oil, optional (it has a
   pungent aroma)

Mix all ingredients in a spray bottle. Shake before use.

Spray into the air but not directly onto furniture or fabrics. Do not spray directly into the eyes. Keep away from children and pets.

Also by Michelle Schoffro Cook, PhD, DNM, ROHP

Print Books

Arthritis-Proof Your Life: The Secret to Pain-Free Living Without Drugs (Humanix)

Be Your Own Herbalist: Over 30 Essential Herbs for Health, Beauty, and Cooking (New World Library)

Boost Your Brain Power in 60 Seconds: The 4-Week Plan for a Sharper Mind, Better Memory, and Healthier Brain (Rodale)

The 4-Week Ultimate Body Detox Plan: A Program for Greater Energy, Health and Vitality (Wiley)

The Probiotic Promise: Simple Steps to Heal Your Body from the Inside Out (DaCapo)

60 Seconds to Slim: Balance Your Body Chemistry to Burn Fat Fast (Rodale)

The Ultimate pH Solution: Balance Your Body Chemistry to Prevent Disease and Lose Weight (HarperCollins)

Weekend Wonder Detox: Quick Cleanses to Strengthen Your Body and Enhance Your Beauty (DaCapo)

E-books

Acid-Alkaline Food Chart

Cancer-Proof: All-Natural Solutions for Cancer-Prevention and Healing

Everything You Need to Know about Healthy Eating

Healing Recipes

The Life Force Diet: 3 Weeks to Supercharge Your Health and Get Slim with Enzyme-Rich Foods

The Phytozyme Cure: Treat or Reverse More than 30 Serious Health Conditions with Powerful Plant Nutrients

Healing Injuries Naturally: How to Mend Bones, Strengthen Joints, Repair Tissue, and Alleviate Pain

Notes

INTRODUCTION

1 "Allergies and Hay Fever," Centers for Disease Control and Prevention, http://www.cdc.gov/nchs/fastats/allergies.htm.
2 Ibid.
3 *Oxford Dictionary*, s.v. "allergy," http://www.oxforddictionaries.com/us/definition/american_english/allergy.

CHAPTER 1

1 Joseph Mercola, DO, "How to Address Allergies and Asthma Symptoms as the 'Worst Allergy Season Ever' Begins," *Mercola.com*, April 18, 2013, http://articles.mercola.com/sites/articles/archive/2013/04/18/allergy-season.aspx.
2 "Fexofenadine Side Effects," *Drugs.com*, http://www.drugs.com/sfx/fexofenadine-side-effects.html.
3 Alan R. Gaby, MD, and the Healthnotes Medical Team, *A-Z Guide to Drug-Herb-Vitamin Interactions*, rev. and exp. 2nd ed. (New York: Three Rivers, 2006), 115–16.
4 "Diphenhydramine Side Effects," *Drugs.com*, http://www.drugs.com/sfx/diphenhydramine-side-effects.html.

5 Gaby and Healthnotes, *A-Z Guide to Drug-Herb-Vitamin Interactions*, 93–94.

6 "Loratadine," *Drugs.com*, http://www.drugs.com/cdi/loratadine .html.

7 Gaby and Healthnotes, *A-Z Guide to Drug-Herb-Vitamin Interactions*, 162.

8 "Cetirizine Side Effects," *Drugs.com*, http://www.drugs.com/ sfx/cetirizine-side-effects.html.

9 Gaby and Healthnotes, *A-Z Guide to Drug-Herb-Vitamin Interactions*, 53–54.

10 Ibid., 104.

11 "Pseudoephedrine Side Effects," *Drugs.com*, http://www .drugs.com/sfx/pseudoephedrine-side-effects.html.

12 "Asthma Treatment: Steroids and Other Anti-Inflammatory Drugs," *WebMD*, http://www.webmd.com/asthma/guide/ asthma-control-with-anti-inflammatory-drugs.

13 "Tests and Procedures: Allergy Shots," Mayo Clinic, http:// www.mayoclinic.org/tests-procedures/allergy-shots/basics/ risks/prc-20014493.

14 Jeffrey S. Bland, *The Disease Delusion: Conquering the Causes of Chronic Illness for a Healthier, Longer, and Happier Life* (New York: Harper Collins, 2014), 39–40.

15 Bahar Gholipour, "Placebo Effect May Account for Half of Drug's Efficacy," *LiveScience*, January 8, 2014, http://www.livescience .com/42430-placebo-effect-half-of-drug-efficacy.html.

16 Bill Sardi, "Does Anybody Still Believe Slam Pieces on Dietary Supplements?," *Orthomolecular Medicine News Service*, August 13, 2012, http://www.orthomolecular.org/resources/ omns/v08n27.shtml.

17 Bland, *The Disease Delusion*, 69.

CHAPTER 2

1 Leslie Ridgway, "High Fructose Corn Syrup Linked to Diabetes," *USC News*, November 28, 2012, https://news.usc.edu/44415/high-fructose-corn-syrup-linked-to-diabetes.

2 Ibid.

3 Ibid.

4 Michelle Schoffro Cook, PhD, DNM, "Monsanto Is Messing with Animals' Sperm," *Care2*, July 24, 2014, http://www.care2.com/greenliving/is-monsanto-making-us-sterile.html.

5 Michelle Schoffro Cook, PhD, DNM, "EPA Classified Roundup as Carcinogen 30 Years Ago . . . but Mysteriously Reversed Decision," *Care2*, March 31, 2015, http://www.care2.com/greenliving/epa-classified-roundup-as-carcinogen-30-years-ago.html.

6 Mark Hyman, MD, "5 Reasons High Fructose Corn Syrup Will Kill You," *DrHyman.com*, http://drhyman.com/blog/2011/05/13/5-reasons-high-fructose-corn-syrup-will-kill-you.

7 Ibid.

8 D. I. Jalal, G. Smits, R. J. Johnson, and M. Chonchol, "Increased Fructose Associates with Elevated Blood Pressure," *Journal of the American Society of Nephrology* 21, no. 9 (September 2010): 1543–49, http://www.ncbi.nlm.nih.gov/pubmed/20595676.

9 Randall Fitzgerald, *The Hundred-Year Lie: How to Protect Yourself from the Chemicals That Are Destroying Your Health* (New York: Penguin, 2006), 72.

10 Ibid., 107.

11 Mandy Oaklander, "7 Side Effects of Drinking Diet Soda," *Prevention*, http://www.prevention.com/food/healthy-eating-tips/diet-soda-bad-you/cell-damage.

12 Ibid.

13 Ibid.

14 Ibid.

15 Betty Kovacs, "Artificial Sweeteners: Health and Disease Prevention," *MedicineNet*, http://www.medicinenet.com/artificial _sweeteners/page5.htm.

16 Joseph Mercola, DO, "Avoiding Artificial Sweeteners? This Study Will Surprise You," September 20, 2011, *Mercola.com*, http://articles.mercola.com/sites/articles/archive/2011/09/ 20/why-are-millions-of-americans-getting-this-synthetic -sweetener-in-their-drinking-water.aspx.

17 S. Bhattacharyya, L. Feferman, T. Unterman, and J. K. Tobacman, "Exposure to Common Food Additive Carrageenan Alone Leads to Fasting Hyperglycemia and in Combination with High Fat Diet Exacerbates Glucose Intolerance and Hyperlipidemia Without Effect on Weight," *Journal of Diabetes Research* (March 25, 2015), http://www.ncbi.nlm.nih.gov/ pubmed/25883986.

18 S. Bhattacharyya, L. Xue, S. Devkota, E. Chang, S. Morris, and J. K. Tobacman, "Carrageenan-Induced Colonic Inflammation Is Reduced in Bcl10 Null Mice and Increased in IL-10-Deficient Mice," *Mediators of Inflammation* (May 26, 2013), http://www.ncbi.nlm.nih.gov/pubmed/23766559.

19 Andrew Weil, MD, "Is Carrageenan Safe?," *DrWeil.com*, October 1, 2012, http://www.drweil.com/drw/u/QAA401181/ Is-Carrageenan-Safe.html.

20 TodayHealth, "Diet Soda Is Doing These 7 Awful Things to Your Body," October 19, 2012, http://www.today.com/health/ diet-soda-doing-these-7-awful-things-your-body-1C6558748.

21 Catherine Paddock, PhD, "Eating Bacon and Hot Dogs Linked to Higher Risk of Lung Disease," *Medical News Today*, April 17, 2007, http://www.medicalnewstoday.com/articles/ 68058.php.

22 James Gallagher, "Process Meat 'Early Death' Link," *BBC*, March 7, 2013, http://www.bbc.co.uk/news/health-21682779.

23 R. Micha, S. K. Wallace, and D. Mozaffarian, "Red and Processed Meat Consumption and Risk of Incident Coronary Heart Disease, Stroke, and Diabetes Mellitus: A Systematic Review and Meta-Analysis," *Circulation* 121, no. 21 (June 1, 2010): 2271–83, http://www.ncbi.nlm.nih.gov/pubmed/20479151.

24 L. A. David, C. F. Maurice, R. N. Carmoday, D. B. Gootenberg, J. E. Button, B. E. Wolfe, A. V. Ling et al., "Diet Rapidly and Reproducibly Alters the Human Gut Microbiome," *Nature* 505, no. 7484 (December 11, 2013): 559–63, http://www.ncbi.nlm.nih.gov/pubmed/24336217.

25 R. Ariano, "Efficacy of a Novel Food Supplement in the Relief of the Signs and Symptoms of Seasonal Allergic Rhinitis and the Reduction of the Consumption of Anti-Allergic Drugs," *Acta BioMedica* 86, no. 1 (April 27, 2015): 53–58, http://www.ncbi.nlm.nih.gov/pubmed/25948028.

26 H. N. Oh, C. E. Kim, J. H. Lee, and J. W. Yang, "Effects of Quercetin in a Mouse Model of Experimental Dry Eye," *Cornea* 34, no. 9 (September 2015): 1130–36, http://www.ncbi.nlm.nih.gov/pubmed/26203745.

27 T. T. Oliveira, K. M. Campos, A. T. Cerqueira-Lima, T. Cana Brasil Carneiro, E. da Silva Velozo, I. C. Ribeiro Melo, E. A. Figueiredo, "Potential Therapeutic Effect of Allium cepa L. and Quercetin in a Murine Model of Blomia tropicalis induced Asthma," *Daru: Journal of the Faculty of Pharmacy, Tehran University of Medical Sciences* 23 (February 21, 2015): 18, http://www.ncbi.nlm.nih.gov/pubmed/25890178.

28 Phyllis A. Balch, *Prescription for Nutritional Healing: A Practical A-to-Z Reference to Drug-Free Remedies* (New York: Avery, 2006).

29 "Food Chart," *Quercetin.com*, http://www.quercetin.com/overview/food-chart.

30 "Apples," World's Healthiest Foods, http://www.whfoods.com/genpage.php?tname=foodspice&dbid=15.

31 Ibid.

CHAPTER 3

1 *Oxford Dictionary*, s.v. "vitamin," http://www.oxfordictionaries
   .com/definition/english/vitamin.

2 "Lynn Margulis Quotes," *BrainyQuote*, http://www.brainyquote
   .com/quotes/quotes/l/lynnmargul495700.html.

3 Xandria Williams, *The Herbal Detox Plan: The Revolutionary
   Way to Cleanse and Revive Your Body* (Carlsbad, CA: Hay
   House, 2004); Gloria Gilbere, "A Doctor's Solution to 'Plumb-
   ing Problems,' in Your Gut That Is!," *Total Health* 26, no. 1
   (February 2004): 37.

4 Leonard Smith, "The Importance of Your Intestinal Tract
   for Health and Longevity," *Townsend Letter: The Examiner of
   Alternative Medicine*, April 2014, 70–72.

5 "4 Steps to Heal Leaky Gut and Autoimmune Disease,"
   DrAxe.com, http://draxe.com/4-steps-to-heal-leaky-gut-and
   -autoimmune-disease.

6 R. J. Bertelsen, A. L. Brantsæter, M. C. Magnus, M. Haugen,
   R. Myhre, B. Jacobsson, M. P. Longnecker et al., "Probiotic
   Milk Consumption in Pregnancy and Infancy and Subsequent
   Childhood Allergic Diseases," *Journal of Allergy and Clinical
   Immunology* 133, no. 1 (January 2014): 165–71, http://www
   .ncbi.nlm.nih.gov/pubmed/24034345.

7 M. Tamura, T. Shikina, T. Morihana, M. Hayama, O. Kajimoto,
   A. Sakamoto, Y. Kajimoto et al., "Effects of Probiotics on Aller-
   gic Rhinitis Induced by Japanese Cedar Pollen: Randomized,
   Double-Blind Placebo-Controlled Clinical Trial," *International
   Archives of Allergy and Immunology* 143, no. 1 (December
   2007): 75–82, http://www.ncbi.nlm.nih.gov/pubmed/17199093.

8 M. A. Moyad, L. E. Robinson, J. M. Kittelsrud, S. G. Reeves,
   S. E. Weaver, A. I. Guzman, and M. E. Bubak, "Immunogenic
   Yeast-Based Fermentation Product Reduces Allergic Rhinitis-
   Induced Nasal Congestion: A Randomized, Double-Blind,

Placebo-Controlled Trial," *Advances in Therapy* 26, no. 8 (August 2009): 795–804, http://www.ncbi.nlm.nih.gov/pubmed/ 19672568.

9 A. W. Nichols, "Probiotics and Athletic Performance: A Systematic Review," *Current Sports Medicine Reports* 6, no. 4 (July 2007): 269–73, http://www.ncbi.nlm.nih.gov/pubmed/ 17618005.

10 H. C. Mei, Y. W. Liu, Y. C. Chiang, S. H. Chao, N. W. Mei, Y. W. Liu, and Y. C. Tsai, "Immunomodulatory Activity of Lactococcus lactis A17 from Taiwan Fermented Cabbage in OVA-Sensitized BALB/c Mice," *Evidence-Based Complementary and Alternative Medicine* (2013), http://www.ncbi.nlm .nih.gov/pubmed/23401710.

11 H. J. Hong, E. Kim, D. Cho, and T. S. Kim, "Differential Suppression of Heat-Killed Lactobacilli Isolated from Kimchi, a Korean Traditional Food, on Airway Hyper-Responsiveness in Mice," *Journal of Clinical Immunology* 30, no. 3 (May 2010): 449–58, http://www.ncbi.nlm.nih.gov/pubmed/20204477.

12 A. M. de Oliveira Leite, M. A. Miguel, R. S. Peixoto, A. S. Rosado, J. T. Silva, and V. M. Paschoalin, "Microbiological, Technological, and Therapeutic Properties of Kefir: A Natural Probiotic Beverage," *Brazilian Journal of Microbiology* 44, no. 2 (October 30, 2013): 341–49, http://www.ncbi.nlm.nih .gov/pubmed/24294220.

13 Y. P. Chen and M. J. Chen, "Effects of Lactobacillus kefiranofaciens M1 Isolated from Kefir Grains on Germ-Free Mice," *PLoS One* 8, no. 11 (November 11, 2013): e78789, http://www .ncbi.nlm.nih.gov/pubmed/24244362.

14 Y. Miyake, S. Sasaki, Y. Ohya, S. Miyamoto, I. Matsunaga, T. Yoshida, Y. Hirota et al., "Soy, Isoflavones, and Prevalence of Allergic Rhinitis in Japanese Women: The Osaka Maternal and Child Health Study," *Journal of Allergy and Clinical Immunology* 115, no. 6 (June 2005): 1176–83, http://www .ncbi.nlm.nih.gov/pubmed/15940131.

15 E. Guillemard, J. Tanguy, A. Flavigny, S. de la Motte, and
    J. Schrezenmeir, "Effects of Consumption of a Fermented Dairy
    Product Containing the Probiotic Lactobacillus casei DN-114
    001 on Common Respiratory and Gastrointestinal Infections
    in Shift Workers in a Randomized Controlled Trial," *Journal
    of the American College of Nutrition* 29, no. 5 (October 2010):
    455–68, http://www.ncbi.nlm.nih.gov/pubmed/21504972.

16 A. Sachdeva, S. Raway, and J. Nagpal, "Efficacy of Fermented
    Milk and Whey Proteins in Helicobacter pylori Eradication:
    A Review," *World Journal of Gastroenterology* 20, no. 3 (Janu-
    ary 21, 2014): 724–37, http://www.ncbi.nlm.nih.gov/pubmed/
    24574746.

17 P. Timan, N. Rojanasthien, M. Manorot, C. Sangdee, and
    S. Teekachunhatean, "Effect of Symbiotic Fermented Milk
    on Oral Bioavailability of Isoflavones in Postmenopausal
    Women," *International Journal of Food Sciences and Nutri-
    tion* 65, no. 6 (September 2014): 761–67, http://www.ncbi
    .nlm.nih.gov/pubmed/24720601.

CHAPTER 4

1   Brian R. Clement, *Living Foods for Optimum Health* (Rose-
    ville, CA: Prima Health, 1998), 39.

2   S. Nakamura, Y. Hashimoto, M. Mikami, E. Yamanaka, T. Soma,
    M. Hino, A. Azuma et al., "Effect of the Proteolytic Enzyme
    Serrapeptase in Patients with Chronic Airway Disease," *Res-
    pirology* 8, no. 3 (September 2003): 316–20, http://www.ncbi
    .nlm.nih.gov/pubmed/12911824.

3   A. H. Swamy Viswanatha and P. A. Patil, "Effect of Some Clin-
    ically Used Proteolytic Enzymes on Inflammation in Rats,"
    Indian Journal of Pharmaceutical Sciences 70, no. 1 (Janu-
    ary 2008): 114–17, http://www.ncbi.nlm.nih.gov/pubmed/
    20390096.

4 D. Gao, Z. Gao, and G. Zhu, "Antioxidant Effects of Lactobacillus plantarum via Activation of Transcription Factor Nrf2,"
Food and Function 4, no. 6 (June 2013): 982–89, http://www
.ncbi.nlm.nih.gov/pubmed/23681127.

CHAPTER 5

1 *Oxford Dictionary*, s.v. "vitamin," http://www.oxforddictionaries
.com/definition/english/vitamin. Emphasis mine.
2 David W. Rowland, *Endocrine Harmony* (Parry Sound, ON:
Health Naturally Publications, 1997), 36–37.
3 Ji Young Choi, Ike Campomayor dela Peña, Seo Young Yoon,
Tae Sun Woo, Yoon Jung Choi, Chan Young Shin, Jong Hoon
et al., "Is the Anti-Stress Effect of Vitamin C Related to Adrenal Gland Function in Rat?," *Food Science & Biotechnology* 20,
no. 2 (April 2011): 429–35, http://link.springer.com/article/
10.1007/s10068-011-0060-3.
4 H. Hemila, "The Effect of Vitamin C on Bronchoconstriction
and Respiratory Symptoms Caused by Exercise: A Review
and Statistical Analysis," *Allergy, Asthma, and Clinical Immunology* 10, no. 1 (November 27, 2014): 58, http://www.ncbi
.nlm.nih.gov/pubmed/25788952.
5 N. E. Lange, D. Sparrow, P. Vokonas, and A. A. Litonjua,
"Vitamin D Deficiency, Smoking, and Lung Function in the
Normative Aging Study," *American Journal of Respiratory
and Critical Care Medicine* 186, no. 7 (October 1, 2012): 616–
21, http://www.ncbi.nlm.nih.gov/pubmed/22822023.
6 E. Shahar, G. Hassoun, and S. Pollack, "Effect of Vitamin E
Supplementation on the Regular Treatment of Seasonal
Allergic Rhinitis," *Annals of Allergy, Asthma, and Immunology* 92, no. 6 (June 2004): 654–58, http://www.ncbi.nlm.nih
.gov/pubmed/15237767.

7 S. Irie, M. Kashiwabara, A. Yamada, and K. Asano, "Suppressive Activity of Quercetin on Periostin Function in Vitro," *In Vivo* 30, no. 1 (January/February 2016): 17–25, http://www.ncbi.nlm.nih.gov/pubmed/26709124.

8 B. Roschek Jr., R. C. Fink, M. McMichael, and R. S. Alberte, "Nettles Extract (Urtica dioica) Affects Key Receptors and Enzymes Associated with Allergic Rhinitis," *Phytotherapy Research* 23, no. 7 (July 2009): 920–26, http://www.ncbi.nlm.nih.gov/pubmed/19140159.

9 H. A. Oh, C. S. Park, H. J. Ahn, Y. S. Park, and H. M. Kim, "Effect of Perilla Frutescens Var. Var Acuta Kudo and Rosmarinic Acid on Allergic Inflammatory Reactions," *Experimental Biology and Medicine* 236, no. 1 (January 2011): 99–106, http://www.ncbi.nlm.nih.gov/pubmed/21239739.

10 T. Makino, Y. Furua, H. Wakushima, H. Jufii, K. Saito, and Y. Kano, "Anti-Allergic Effect of Perilla Frutescens and Its Active Constituents," *Phytotherapy Research* 17, no. 3 (March 2003): 240–43, http://www.ncbi.nlm.nih.gov/pubmed/12672153.

11 J. C. Heo, D. Y. Nam, M. S. Seo, and S. H. Lee, "Alleviation of Atopic Dermatitis-Related Symptoms by Perilla Frutescens Britton," *International Journal of Molecular Medicine* 28, no. 5 (November 2011): 733–37, http://www.ncbi.nlm.nih.gov/pubmed/21811759.

12 W. W. Ji, R. P. Li, M. Li, S. Y. Wang, X. Zhang, X. X. Niu, W. Li et al., "Antidepressant-Like Effect of Essential Oil of Perilla Frutescens in Chronic, Unpredictable, Mild Stress-Induced Depression Model Mice," *Chinese Journal of Natural Medicine* 12, no. 10 (October 2014): 753–59, http://www.ncbi.nlm.nih.gov/pubmed/25443368.

13 R. Guo, M. H. Pittler, and E. Ernst, "Herbal Medicines for the Treatment of Allergic Rhinitis: A Systematic Review," *Annals of Allergy, Asthma, and Immunology* 99, no. 6 (December 2007): 483–95, http://www.ncbi.nlm.nih.gov/pubmed/18219828.

14 A. Brattström, A. Schapowal, I. Maillet, B. Schnyder, B. Ryffel, and R. Moser, "Petasites Extract ze339 (PET) Inhibits Allergy-Induced Th2 Responses, Airway Inflammation and Airway Hyperreactivity in Mice," *Phytotherapy Research* 24, no. 5 (May 2010): 680–85, http://www.ncbi.nlm.nih.gov/pubmed/19827027.

15 A. Schapowol and Petasites Study Group, "Randomised Control Trial of Butterbur and Cetirizine for Treating Seasonal Allergic Rhinitis," *BMJ* 324, no. 7330 (January 19, 2002): 144–46, http://www.ncbi.nlm.nih.gov/pubmed/11799030.

16 D. J. Kwon, Y. S. Bae, S. M. Ju, A. R. Goh, G. S. Youn, S. Y. Choi, and J. Park, "Casuarinin Suppresses TARC/CCL17 and MDC/CCL22 Production via Blockade of NF-kB and STAT1 Activation in HaCaT Cells," *Biochemical and Biophysical Research Communications* 417, no. 4 (January 27, 2012): 1254–59, http://www.ncbi.nlm.nih.gov/pubmed/22227193.

CHAPTER 8

1 Alison Cohen, Sarah Janssen, MD, PhD, MPH, and Gina Solomon, MD, MPH, "Clearing the Air: Hidden Hazards of Air Fresheners," *NRDC*, September 2007, http://www.nrdc.org/health/home/airfresheners/airfresheners.pdf.

2 C. G. Bornehag, J. Sundell, C. J. Weschler, T. Sigsgaard, B. Lundgren, M. Hasselgren, and L. Hägerhed-Engman, "The Association Between Asthma and Allergic Symptoms in Children and Pthalates in House Dust: A Nested, Case-Control Study," *Environmental Health Perspectives* 112, no. 14 (October 2004): 1393–97, http://www.ncbi.nlm.nih.gov/pubmed/15471731.

3 Cohen, Janssen, and Solomon, "Clearing the Air."

4 Jason Tchir, "How Many Car Air Fresheners Are Too Many?," *Globe and Mail*, August 13, 2013, http://www.theglobeandmail.com/globe-drive/culture/commuting/how-many-car-air-fresheners-are-too-many/article13727443.

5   "Greener School Cleaning Supplies: School Cleaner Test Results,"
    EWG, November 3, 2009, http://www.ewg.org/research/greener
    -school-cleaning-supplies/school-cleaner-test-results.

6   "Air Fresheners," *SilentMenace.com*, http://www.silentmenace
    .com/-Air_Fresheners_.html.

7   "8 Household Cleaning Agents to Avoid," *Gaiam*, http://life
    .gaiam.com/article/8-household-cleaning-agents-avoid.

8   Ibid.

9   "Does Vinegar Kill Germs?," David Suzuki Foundation, http://
    davidsuzuki.org/what-you-can-do/queen-of-green/faqs/
    cleaning/does-vinegar-kill-germs.

10 "8 Household Cleaning Agents to Avoid."

11 Ibid.

12 Ibid.

13 Ibid.

14 Kurt Schnaubelt, PhD, *Advanced Aromatherapy: The Science of
    Essential Oil Therapy* (Rochester, VT: Healing Arts, 1995), 35.

15 "Tea Tree," *MateriaAromatica.com*, http://materiaaromatica
    .com/Default.aspx?go=Article&ArticleID=225.

16 "EWG Cleaners Database—Hall of Shame," *EWG*, 2012,
    http://static.ewg.org/reports/2012/cleaners_hallofshame/
    cleaners_hallofshame.pdf.

17 "Volkswagen's U.S. Emissions Settlement Will Reportedly
    Cost $15 Billion," *Fortune*, June 28, 2016, http://fortune.com/
    2016/06/28/volkswagen-emissions-settlement.

18 "Diesel Engines and Public Health," Union of Concerned
    Scientists, http://www.ucsusa.org/clean_vehicles/why-clean
    -cars/air-pollution-and-health/trucks-buses-and-other
    -commercial-vehicles/diesel-engines-and-public.html#
    .VyEiV3pOLOR.

19 Ibid.

20 Daniel Moore, MD, "Capsaicin for Nasal Symptoms," *Verywell*,
    http://www.verywell.com/capsaicin-for-nasal-symptoms
    -82769.

Resources

AROMATHERAPY AND HERBAL SUPPLIES

THERE ARE SOME EXCELLENT companies that offer dried or bulk herbs for use in your aromatherapy oils and creams or herbs for teas. Two of my favorite suppliers are

Harmonic Arts

Harmonic Arts offers a wide range of herbs, natural foods, and some amazing medicinal herb blends. Yarrow and Angela Willard, the founders of Harmonic Arts, also offer many instructional and entertaining videos worth checking out on their site.
https://harmonicarts.ca

Mountain Rose Herbs

Mountain Rose Herbs offers a range of herbs and aromatherapy products worth checking out.
http://www.mountainroseherbs.com

Index

About the Author

Michelle Schoffro Cook, PhD, DNM, DHS, ROHP, is the author of twenty health books, including *Arthritis-Proof Your Life* and the international best-sellers *60 Seconds to Slim*, *The Ultimate pH Solution*, and *The 4-Week Ultimate Body Detox Plan*. Her books have been translated into many languages, including Spanish, Greek, Chinese, Thai, Indonesian, and Russian. She holds advanced degrees in natural health, holistic and ortho-molecular nutrition, and traditional natural medicine, and she has twenty-five years of experience in the field. Dr. Cook is a board-certified doctor of natural medicine who has received the Doctor of Humanitarian Services designation from the World Organization of Natural Medicine and a World-Leading Intellectual Award for her contribution to natural medicine. She is a regular blogger for CulturedCook.com and Care2.com. She owns her own food consultancy company known as PureFood BC, which offers strategic management, marketing and communications services. Visit her websites: DrMichelleCook.com, PureFoodBC.com, and WorldsHealthiestDiet.com.

World's Healthiest News

You can subscribe to Dr. Schoffro Cook's free e-zine, *World's Healthiest News*, to obtain natural health insights, news, research, recipes, and more. Each edition features natural approaches to boost your energy, supercharge your immune system, and look and feel great. Subscribe at: WorldsHealthiestDiet.com.

Dr. Cook's Blogs

Don't miss a single blog by Dr. Cook! Follow her at:

DrMichelleCook.com
CulturedCook.com
HealthySurvivalist.com
Care2.com/GreenLiving/author/MCook

E-Books

Discover Dr. Cook's exclusive e-books on her site:
WorldsHealthiestDiet.com
Follow her on:

Twitter @mschoffrocook
Facebook facebook.com/drschoffrocook
Pinterest pinterest.com/drmichellecook